Don't Die of Embarrassment

LIFE AFTER COLOSTOMY
AND OTHER ADVENTURES

Barbara Barrie

Afterword by
Dr. Otis W. Brawley

A FIRESIDE BOOK
PUBLISHED BY SIMON & SCHUSTER

FIRESIDE
Rockefeller Center
1230 Avenue of the Americas
New York, NY 10020

First Fireside Edition 1999

FIRESIDE and colophon are registered trademarks of Simon & Schuster Inc.

DESIGNED BY ERICH HOBBING

Set in Palatino

Manufactured in the United States of America

10 9 8 7 6 5 4 3 2 1

Library of Congress Cataloging-in-Publication Data
Barrie, Barbara.
    [Second act]
    Don't die of embarrassment : life after colostomy and other adventures /
Barbara Barrie ; afterword by Otis W. Brawley.
        p. cm.
    Includes index.
    1. Barrie, Barbara—Health. 2. Rectum—Cancer—Patients—United States—
Biography. 3. Colostomy—Popular works. 4. Actresses—United States—
Biography. I. Title.
RC280.R37B37 1999
362.1'9699435'0092—dc21
[B]   98-52468
                                                                           CIP

ISBN 0-684-84624-1

"Season," from *The Vixen* by W. S. Merwin, © 1995 by W. S. Merwin. Reprinted by
permission of Alfred A. Knopf, Inc.

The names of some of the individuals in this book have been changed.

Originally published as *Second Act: Life After Colostomy and Other Adventures*

Acknowledgments

My word processor has always been a semi-enemy, and there have been countless occasions when my friend Judy Rich has run to my side to get me out of whatever trouble has reared its horrible head. One day she had to suffer my putting my head upon her shoulder and sobbing after she recovered a chapter I thought I had erased forever. Without her visits and our endless phone conversations, both of us with our computers turned on as she nursed me through a procedure, I could not have written this book.

My longtime friend and agent, George Nicholson, has been enthusiastic about this project since the day I first mentioned it to him. And he is the world's greatest laugher.

Jane Rosenman, my amazing editor, led me into paths of writing I didn't think possible, and Jill Feldman, her talented assistant, has been my "phone pal" on all aspects of *Second Act*. They made me feel like a member of a really good team.

The first person to see a word of my manuscript was a new friend, the wonderful writer Natalie Robins. From that initial faxed page, she has been wildly encouraging and supportive. She has been one of the "gifts" of my disease.

Karen Recca, my oncologist's secretary, has put up with my canceling, forgetting, and changing appointments for over two years. She has a direct, kind way of dealing with all of Dr. Mears's patients, and I have always wondered how she manages to do it with such grace.

Acknowledgments

I salute all the medical people everywhere who have aided me along the way—the maintenance teams, the nurses, the IV specialists, the drivers, the gurney pushers, the radiation technicians. Many of them are discussed in the book, but unfortunately I can't mention them all personally.

And, of course, I thank all my friends and family who have made this journey with me.

For Jay, Jane, and Aaron
and for Terry Haus

Contents

Contents

Don't Die of Embarrassment

I am very excited to see more of India. There are so many people here, and the lifestyles and cultures are so diverse. The dense population forces one to change his concept of numbers. It influences every activity, from fighting for a seat on a bus, to waiting in line at an Indian cinema (a truly unique adventure), to weaving through bicycle traffic jams at rush hour. Religious festivals are seen constantly, for almost every day of the year a Hindu god is being celebrated somewhere in India. The colors, smells, sounds, and unique atmosphere make a part of every day an adventure.

A quote from athlete and writer TIM O'CONNELL, whose 1988 tour took him, by bicycle, from the Arctic Circle to Egypt. He was an ostomate from the age of two.

CHAPTER 1

New Beginnings

I have a deep, unreasonable desire to own a picture by William Merritt Chase, the American artist who painted scenes of eastern Long Island: the shimmering blue-black ponds; beautiful children in white dresses playing in the sand, their mothers sitting on blankets, ruffled parasols held over their heads to protect them from the golden sun of an August afternoon.

These magical people, I know, will go home to their shingled houses and have lobster salad on blue-ceilinged porches, their wicker chairs cushioned in gingham, pots of geraniums tucked into dappled corners. Later, in the early evening, the fathers will play croquet with the children on emerald lawns, and the mothers will read stories to them in their cool beds.

I used to long to be part of those pictures. Probably because, as a girl in Texas, I dropped ragged kitchen string for crab into the Bay of Corpus Christi, Texas, ate them with my fingers from paper plates, and lived in a cramped tourist-court apartment with tumbledown Grand Rapids furniture. My father worked as an insurance salesman late into the steaming Texas nights. My clothes were hand-me-downs from relatives in Chicago, and the smell of must and mildew was deeply imbedded in everything we touched.

Is it any wonder that I love William Merritt Chase?

Occasionally there is a canvas for sale at a Madison

Avenue gallery, and I will abandon my blue jeans and sneakers and don a decent dress and shoes (so that the receptionist won't sneer at me). I'll even put on mascara and lipstick and change my nylon knapsack for a leather purse and visit the gallery. I will become a proper white-haired lady who just *might* be a prospective customer. I could never afford such a painting, of course, but at least I can go and visit it.

I'll tiptoe across the marble floors to find the canvas. There, in its ornate, slightly dulled gold frame, is the summer light, the play of mashed-potato clouds billowing over spiny beach grass, the Atlantic Ocean breaking in shallow, even waves on the shore.

My husband, Jay, knows about this William Merritt Chase passion. My kids, Aaron and Jane, also know. When they were little, they always complained each time I dragged them to the Metropolitan Museum of Art, or the Frick, or the Museum of Modern Art. But Aaron soon loved the Frick (all those people in funny hats on festooned garden swings), and Jane fell under the spell of Cézanne, Monet, and Renoir. In 1994 she flew home on the Red Eye from Los Angeles just to see the Origins of Impressionism exhibit at the Met. Sometimes parenting pays off. Sometimes.

In 1954 I was a struggling young actress, living in a cold-water flat (that means hot water, but no heat) on Second Avenue in Manhattan. One day, after the sudden, unexpected demise of a love affair, I found myself so depressed that I was unable to rise from my bed, where I was found one day at three in the afternoon.

"Barbara, I can't believe you're not up yet." It was Mark Rydell, a director-actor friend phoning me from his set.

"I know." My body was wound in the sheets, my lips were almost glued together. "I can't move."

"You know, Barbara, it's not about this guy. He represents some fucking thing in your life, in your childhood. . . ."

I started to weep. "I'm sure of it, Mark, but I just can't seem to recover."

"Yes, you can. You're talking to the world's champion analysand. Twelve years is record-setting, wouldn't you say?"

"Right."

"Get up right now. Drink some coffee. I'm going to phone someone and make an appointment for you. I'll call you right back."

Two days later I began an eight-year Freudian analysis with Dr. Joseph Levy, a rotund, genial doctor who had fled Hitler's Germany in the late 1930s.

Dr. Levy's office, on East 81st Street, was across the street from the Metropolitan Museum of Art, and I'd hop in almost daily to see an exhibit, just wander around, have a cup of tea, still in the haze of the session I'd just finished.

In those days there was practically no one in the museum. I'm not exaggerating. I had the echoing galleries and the broad marble staircase to myself. The guards knew me, and I knew them.

"How are you today?" a guard would ask, grateful for someone to talk to.

"Fine," I'd say. Little did he know that I had just spent the last hour sobbing my heart out or railing at poor Dr. Levy for a hundred different eight-year-old's reasons.

Today, an amber October afternoon in 1993, throngs of people bustled about in their casual clothes. Young couples pushing baby carriages, older people in their exercise suits, art students in head-to-toe black, sitting on the floor and sketching or making notes. People with backpacks, Mark Cross purses, running shoes, long skirts, shorts, torn T-shirts, Valentino coats.

I had gone to see an exhibit of American painters at the Metropolitan. Mainly, of course, because of Chase and because of J. Alden Weir, another American whose paintings were being shown. The homeliness of his landscapes and portraits is, to me, unrealistically, my own secret discovery.

I had a serene early lunch in the cafeteria and then wandered through the collection. I was in hog heaven, as we say in Texas—listening to Philippe de Montebello's mellifluous voice speak to me through the earphones of the programmed cassette I had rented.

At four-fifteen I reluctantly left the museum. Practically running across Central Park, I just made a five o'clock aerobics class at the gym on 76th Street and Broadway, where I jumped about like a mad person, lifted weights, pushed against rubber bands wrapped around my legs, and dissolved into a pool of sweat. It felt wonderful. More wonderful when it was over, but I had to keep the fat at bay and the heart rate up, didn't I?

On to Fairway Market, at Broadway and 74th Street, for vegetables and fruit for dinner. The rest of the West Side was shopping there too. It's always bedlam. The cheery manager, Heshie Hochman, okayed my check.

"So Barbara," he said, "what's happening with the career?"

"The usual, Hesh. Just did a Movie of the Week in North Carolina, and I'm back now working on my book."

"You got another book coming out?" He held out his hand. "You want me to okay your check?"

"Yes, thanks."

"What's it about?" he asked, scribbling his initials on the check.

"It's about a kid with dyslexia and how he learns to read."

"Oh, yeah, you know, my sister's kid had that. It's rough."

"It's very rough," I said.

"Well, good luck, darling. I want to read that book when you finish it." He gave me a sweet kiss on the cheek and patted my shoulder. "Consuelo, the check's okay," he shouted over the din of impatient shoppers, market carts, and cash registers.

The heavy plastic bags made red-ribbon indentations on my palms, and I stopped at Broadway and 72nd to allow the blood to flow again. The apartment buildings loomed like black kindergarten-cutouts against the orange six o'clock sky. The treetops at Riverside Park were little green dots, barely visible, like the quick, eloquent brush strokes of William Merritt Chase's Southampton trees.

When I entered our apartment a few minutes later, the living room was glowing with the last of the light. We live twenty-seven floors up, facing the west side of Manhattan, the Hudson River, New Jersey, and of course the sunsets. Jay, my husband, says you can see the sun go down, but you can never see even one light pop on in any building. He's right. We have sat, vodkas in hand, and fruitlessly searched for one window to turn yellow. Only the gremlins and fairies can see that.

The message machine was blinking. Four insistent blinks. I listened: call Wendy Lamb, your editor at Doubleday; call your husband, your daughter, and Scott Landis at Innovative Artists.

I called Scott, my gangly, smart young agent.

"Barbara, I'm glad you caught me. How are you?"

"Great. How's your banker girlfriend?"

"Oh, it's over, I'm afraid."

"Oh, Scott, I'm so sorry."

"Yeah, well . . ." He caught his breath, cleared his throat. "Listen, I have an interesting offer for you."

Hey, this was good news. "A firm offer?"

"Oh, yes. CBS. It's *Scarlett*, the sequel to *Gone with the Wind*, you know. An eight-hour mini-series."

"Who's directing?"

I could hear him shifting in his chair. "Sally, will you hand me that breakdown sheet? Thanks. Let's see. It's John Erman."

"Oh, John," I yelled. "I love to work with John."

"I know you do. He wants you and Elizabeth Wilson to play Scarlett's two aunts. It's two trips to London around Christmas and then a break. Then Charleston in the spring."

"Elizabeth?" I started walking around in excitement— thanks to the portable phone. "Oh, she's a mad, wonderful thing. We've been friends for thirty years, but we've never worked together. This is a dream. Do you think it will happen?"

Scott was practically grinning over the telephone. "Why not? It's a good deal, if you want to do it."

"Have you read the script?"

"Yes. It's not a big part, but you're seen a lot. If you're interested, I'll send it over by messenger in the morning."

London! Charleston! I'd never been to Charleston. "Of course I'm interested." Interested? I was almost jumping up and down. "Oh, how about the money?" I asked.

"We're still negotiating," he said, still sounding pleased, "but it'll be very, very nice."

"How splendid. Shouldn't I do it?"

"The only problem, Barbara, is the in-between time. About three months. They won't pay you for that, but they'll pay a lot for the time you do work. And it's first-class travel and hotel and a trailer of your own . . . all that stuff. Yes, I think you ought to do it. You'll have a ball."

"What a great gig. What could be bad?"

"You may even owe me a lunch for this, Barbara."

"Anywhere. Any time. Just name your place."

"How about Lutèce?"

"Lutèce?"

"Just kidding."

I sighed a loud imitation sigh. "Thank God."

"How about the Carnegie Deli?"

"You're on, Scott."

"Okay, lunch is settled. Oh, and the billing will be worked out later, probably alphabetical, after the big stars."

"Sounds good," I said.

"And here's the last bit of news: You have scenes with Sir John Gielgud."

Now I sat down hard on Jay's leather chair. "I'll take it! I'll take it!"

Jay came home from his rehearsal, and we took our drinks to the window seat, turned off the lights, and watched the sky go deep blue, then almost black. (No, we didn't see one light come on—they all just gradually, mysteriously appeared.)

"How was the exhibit, Barbara?"

"Oh, fabulous, just incredible."

"Did you buy a William Merritt Chase?"

"Yes, two of them."

"Good. I'll send the check tomorrow." My husband is a very droll man.

"Wouldn't it be amazing to have one hanging here in the living room, Jay?"

"My darling, if I were a millionaire, I would buy you every one that's for sale."

"I know you would."

We sat quietly for a while. I told him about the offer for *Scarlett*.

"How terrific. Are you going to do it?"

"I can't think why not. It would certainly pay some bills right now."

"Amen," he said.

"And if I'm in London, you could visit and we could go to the theater and the opera."

"And you could go to the Harrod's Christmas sale."

"Where I could afford to buy one tie and one sweater."

"But you could at least be there, Barb."

"And we could go back to Sir John Soane's museum."

Jay sat up straight. "It would be a good time to see some children's theater . . . Christmas, the pantomimes, all that."

"Oh, Jay, it'll be such a treat. Shall we ask Jane and Aaron if they want to join us?"

"Don't get carried away until everything's worked out, Barbara." That's what Jay always says about these things. He's the artistic director of Theatreworks/USA, a foundation that produces original plays and musicals for children. "First, let's see if you get an extra ticket with the deal and how much money you're really getting."

Two weeks later the contracts were signed and the airline

tickets were in my desk drawer. During November and early December I tried to finish our new apartment. We had moved that year from our huge, old apartment on West End Avenue, and the painters and electricians were just finishing up.

There were still many things to do, a punch-list for the contractor: a kitchen light that didn't work, a loose door-knob, shelves to be installed.

I had to be examined by the *Scarlett* doctor, to be sure I was healthy and insurable. Deciding to lose a little weight for the filming, I stepped up exercise classes and ran an extra mile or so in Central Park every other day.

Each morning I set aside four hours to work on my book, but that's always hard. When I'm supposed to sit down at the computer, I can find so many other absolutely necessary things to do: clean drawers, read W. S. Merwin poetry, make a tuna salad for dinner, write a thank-you note, call the children in California . . . anything to keep from working. And now, of course, I had to find out what would be happening in London and Charleston. I had a lot of essential travel reading to do, didn't I?

Whatever excursion we took when Aaron and Jane were kids and however disastrous or wonderful it was, I always used to say, "It's an adventure. Consider it an adventure."

Well, now I was going off to work with John Gielgud. And run my mile each day in Hyde Park. Be with my family in gray, glorious London. Shop, go to the Tate Gallery, eat Indian food in every other corner restaurant of the city. This was going to be an adventure.

CHAPTER 2

London

In December I went to London for costume fittings, wig fittings, rehearsals, and general introduction to the production.

First class on British Air: footrests, champagne, one's own tiny television screen with a vast choice of films from which to choose, nighttime eyeshades and blue slippers, and two-piece pajamas. I couldn't get over that—pajamas. It doesn't matter how many times I've traveled like this over the years, it's always such fun—like playing grown-up when you know, deep down, you're still a kid.

I had two rooms high above Hyde Park: one for Aaron and one for Jay and me. They would be following later, after all the preliminary preparation was done. Jane was working and in the midst of a serious romance in Los Angeles and had decided not to join us.

"Mom, I wish I could be with you, but really, I can't always be the little child following you around."

"I know, darling, you have your own life."

"Yes, exactly."

"But maybe you could come for just a few days."

"*Mom!* What did we just say?"

"I know, I know. I have to let go. But you adore London . . ."

"*Mom!*"

I am a terrible mother. They write Movies of the Week about people like me.

The production company whisked the actors around London in limousines from one appointment to another. There were flowers and notes of welcome in the rooms, people rushing to open doors, costume assistants bringing bottled water or little biscuits into the fitting rooms. I just loved it all.

Elizabeth Wilson arrived a day later, wheeling into the lobby with her perfectly packed bags, her chiffon scarf fluttering over her beautiful brown hair, her complexion rosy, glowing, wrinkle-less, with mini-series people and two bell-men streaming behind her.

On a rainy day the next week, with the anemones poking up in vivid masses everywhere in London, Jay and Aaron arrived. Because the actors didn't work every day, we had time to go to museums, to the National Theatre at night, and to little restaurants in the neighborhood of our hotel . . . one, alas, where Aaron contracted violent food poisoning and then spent the next six days in bed under the care of a wildly expensive physician: cravat, little round spectacles, beard and all.

"I am never never leaving the United States again as long as I live," he said, after throwing up for two days. Who could blame him?

Not long after that Jay came down with the flu and was surrounded by nose drops, bunched-up tissues, and a vaporizer obtained from the hotel housekeeping department.

I brought in meals from Shepherd's Market, which was right in back of the hotel. I ran out constantly to replenish the Coke and juice supply. I bathed Aaron's head in wet cloths. I rubbed Jay's back and begged him not to snore. I cleaned up the bathrooms at least twice a day and changed Aaron's linens constantly, he was so drenched with fever. In our room I held Jay's hand while he moaned and tried to nap.

I wanted to kill them both.

Meanwhile we were rehearsing in an old mansion, with a circular driveway, a few blocks from the hotel. The rehearsal table was long and ancient, and the paneled walls had been mirrored over in twentieth-century glass that cheapened the gracious room. But one could imagine the glorious balls and feasts and weddings that had taken place in this building, the music playing, the vases overflowing with lush flower arrangements. Only by looking carefully could I see the cigarette burns in the carpet, the scraped paint along the baseboards, the fluorescent tubing where once had hung dazzling, ornate chandeliers.

In a separate room were coffee machines and tea urns, sandwiches and cakes, where, when we were not needed, we could visit with the other actors, many of whom were English and Irish.

George Grizzard, a very dear friend, was playing Scarlett's lawyer. He and Elizabeth Wilson had performed together in many plays for more than twenty years. They fell into each other's arms.

"Where are you staying, Liz?"

"At your hotel . . . we're all there, didn't you know?"

"How's your room?" he asked her.

She waved her long, willowy arms in the air. "My dear, I'm just so thrilled to be here, they could put me in a closet and I wouldn't say a word."

The first day, Elizabeth and I rehearsed two scenes with Joanne Whalley-Kilmer, who was playing Scarlett. She is a surprisingly tiny girl, considering the fact that as we were introduced, she was finishing a Big Mac, french fries with catsup, and a milk shake. She wore no makeup; her face was clear and honest.

And she was very talented. Obviously her preparation was extensive, as she had already been working with John Erman for two weeks before we arrived. Clever, sharp, stubborn, sexy Scarlett was already sitting in the chair and talking to us.

After the first read-through, John carefully explained our family relationships and the "back story" of these characters: who had been our ancestors, how Scarlett ended up in America, and the mores and manners of the times. I panicked.

Why hadn't *I* done more preparation? Shouldn't I know all this?

"Remember, Barbara, you and Elizabeth are the poor relations. Your income is practically nonexistent, so you are very dependent on the good graces of Sir John." We were all on a break; steaming cups of tea, biscuits, and crackers had been placed on the table. Joanne Whalley-Kilmer was eating another Big Mac.

"Was I ever married?" I asked. (Many actors speak of their character as "I," rather than "she" or "he." Speaking in the first person lessens the distance between ourselves and the people we are playing.)

"Yes, you could have been," replied John. "You were in the book, I think."

"Oh, right," I said. "I forgot."

"Would you like to be?"

"I think so. A little less clichéd than the two spinster sisters, don't you think?" (I hoped that I sounded really thoughtful here.)

"Absolutely. We'll get you a little gold ring."

"Very modest, John."

"Oh, darling . . . really modest."

"Do you suppose I had children, even though they weren't mentioned in the story?"

"No, that's why you're so attached to Scarlett. She's your dead sister's child. She's the young person in your life."

We rehearsed both scenes again. This time it was easier, thanks to John's background research and specific, detailed direction.

Elizabeth and I began to develop a sisterlike symbiosis. We had never worked together, and this process was like meeting a totally new person. By the time we "wrapped" in London, we had exchanged stories about our entire lives, about former lovers, hated directors, beloved directors, horrible movie shoots, happy and unhappy runs on Broadway.

She was so enchanting, so quirky, and so amazingly kind

to everyone. And she did things only in her own way. When she had spent enough time at an art exhibit, she would say, "Well, dear, I've just had enough. I want to go back to the hotel, and I'm going. You just stay and have a lovely time. I'll see you tomorrow."

"Do you want to have dinner, Liz, later?"

"Oh, no, thanks, honey, I have a few little things in my room, and I'll just eat them and go to sleep early. Besides, I want to work on the script." And out of the museum she would sail, listing slightly to the side to compensate for a troublesome knee.

The first rehearsal was over. For the rest of the week we would be working here; then location shooting, all around London, would begin in two or three days. As we were all gathering our scripts and raincoats and water bottles, John smiled like a proud father. "Girls, girls, it's going to be wondrous."

"From your lips to God's ear," I said, grateful that we had leapt the hurdle of the first day. Jeanne Moreau was once quoted as saying that she always wanted to destroy the first day's shooting of every film. Her acting, she felt, was always unrelaxed in the beginning, as she wasn't yet comfortable with her new colleagues. Any actor will tell you how exactly right she was: The first day is usually awkward and tortuous.

"Joanne, you are just fabulous," said Elizabeth, as she folded her silk scarf into the neck of her trench coat.

"Thank you, really, thank you. I've always admired you both so much. It's a thrill to be working with you."

A lovely, well-mannered girl. And an Acting Force.

Early the next week Sir John Gielgud arrived for rehearsal. We were all very nervous. Could we actually sit down and *act* with this man whom we had idolized for years? I was paralyzed with the usual actor's dilemma: Now they'll really find out I have no talent. They'll do my scene with Sir John and decide they made an appalling mistake and send me back to New York.

We had been drinking our afternoon tea, and when he was ushered in, everyone in the room stood up and practically genuflected to this extraordinary man, full of charm and dignity. He was amazingly tall and elegant, pink-cheeked and very shy. We all quickly realized that he was not interested in small talk. He wanted to work, and that's what we did.

We sat around the table and rehearsed a dinner scene that included Joanne Whalley-Kilmer, Elizabeth, Sir John, and me. It was a funny scene, in which Sir John is given a birthday cake, and Joanne, as Scarlett, is fairly impudent to her imperious grandfather.

After a low-keyed first reading, Sir John looked at our director and said thoughtfully, "I think, John dear, that the birthday cake will be very important. I think I can do quite a good deal with it, don't you?"

We all laughed. Of course he would do a lot with the birthday cake. He would probably make a brilliant scenario of cutting and eating the cake while dealing with these difficult women (and that is exactly what he did about a month later in a crumbling dowager of a country house, an hour from London, where we shot all the "grandfather scenes").

Finally he stood up. We all rose instantly. Bowing slightly, he shook hands with each person and murmured how delighted he was to be working with us. Placing a careful hand under Sir John's elbow, his assistant steered him out of the room and down the winding staircase. Rehearsal was over.

Carl Reiner had once said to me (about the longevity of his career), "I'm just waiting until they find out."

Well, I had rehearsed with John Gielgud, and they hadn't found out.

Yet.

CHAPTER 3

Charleston

Charleston that morning was hot. The pastel houses shimmered in the early-morning sun. I looked out the window of my air-conditioned trailer, with its stenciled walls and Early American upholstery. Breakfast burritos, cereal, pancakes, bagels, coffee, and juice were being served to the crew and to actors in nineteenth-century waistcoats and britches, hoop skirts and bonnets—a crazy contrast to the cables and lighting equipment and trucks in the parking lot where we were all encamped.

It was April 1994, four months after I had finished the work in London.

The *Scarlett* company was completing a "market" sequence on the campus of the University of Charleston, a few blocks away. The art department had built a flower-filled, vegetable-laden series of stalls, which this morning was a noisy, busy place where Julie Harris and Jean Smart were in the last few minutes of their scene.

After that we were scheduled to move around the corner to a large house where Elizabeth Wilson, Joanne Whalley-Kilmer, and I were to do a "drive-up" scene, and there Julie Harris would meet us at the gate. The horse and carriage were waiting in the heat, and Elizabeth and I, in elaborate wigs, heavy corsets, and layers of petticoats, were ensconced in our trailers.

I have learned that a nine o'clock "on set" call usually

means that you will start working around eleven o'clock, if you're lucky. If not, you can wait all day to utter perhaps two lines in a small scene and then get sent home at "wrap time" not having set foot anywhere near the location or sound-stage. It's called "Hurry up and wait," and all film actors are familiar with it.

So this morning I closed the window and sat down at my laptop computer. I was almost at the end of my young-adult book, going over, word by word, the notes from the copy reader. The publisher was talking to cover artists, and after tortuous discussions, the title was now to be *Adam Zigzag.*

Over my petticoats I wore a long man's shirt, and my feet were bare. The coffeepot was warm in the little galley kitchen, and on the radio I had the local classical music station. My makeup, finished at eight o'clock, only needed a little touch-up, and the taffeta dress and bonnet were on hangers hooked over the closet door.

After another hour, a knock on the door. "Miss Barrie, we're ten minutes away from you," said the second A.D. (assistant director). "One more shot in this scene." That usually means another hour, but I said, "Fine. Will you please send someone to help me dress?"

Our costume designer, Marit Allen, tapped on the door. "Good morning, Barbara dear. Time to get into the robes?" she asked in her lovely British accent. She climbed up the steep metal stairs and sank for a moment on the banquette. "My word, it's hot out there. You must be very careful today in all this stuff. Drink lots of water and let us know if anything is too tight or uncomfortable."

Marit was stunning and fresh. Who else would have the nerve to combine tight blue jeans with a Chinese kimono and cowboy boots? Her hair was pulled up in back with a tortoiseshell barrette, and her long, shiny earrings sparkled in the light. She slipped the dress over my head. "Breathe in . . . oh yes, a bit loose, do you think? Oh, well, never mind. The little jacket will cover it."

I sat down while she laced up the boots. Real clunkers. I couldn't have done it myself: The corset wouldn't allow me to bend over. No wonder all those long-ago women had maids. Then she placed the bonnet on my wig and tied the bow beneath my chin as only a professional can do. It was perfect. I was now ready to work, if only they would call me.

An hour and a half later, they did. The A.D. helped me down the steps while I held up the huge skirt. "Sorry, Miss Barrie. Hope you weren't in the costume too long."

"Not at all, thank you." I have learned not to complain about anything—it isn't worth it. As my husband says about acting, "Say the words, don't bump into the furniture, and *get off!*"

But now something funny was happening. I suddenly couldn't see too clearly. My peripheral vision was dancing a tango, and the pink and yellow buildings seemed to be undulating into the sidewalk. I was amazingly dizzy. I stopped to clear my head as the A.D. grabbed my elbow.

"Miss Barrie, are you okay?" he asked.

"Yes, just a little blinded by the light." But I was terribly nauseated. Had that ritzy restaurant last night served me a slightly aged swordfish?

"Your makeup will be touched up on the set," he said.

"Fine. Can I walk there?"

"Yes, but the van is waiting. Maybe you should hop a ride."

"No, no. It would do me more good to walk. Just point me in the right direction."

The location was just around the corner, a block and a half away. I walked along The Battery, which skirts the historic Charleston Bay, and at a lush park I turned right and headed toward the white-columned house. Bystanders were watching as the lighting equipment was being set up and the extras were rehearsing. I was having trouble focusing, but I was certainly not going to tell anyone. The show must go on, mustn't it?

It was now almost noon. The dress was clinging in taffeta ripples to my back, and waves of heat snaked across the street, which had been covered with gravel and dirt to look as it did in 1840. John Erman, his handsome face smiling and secure, turned to me as I approached his chair.

"Hi, dear. Are you ready for your big moment?"

"Absolutely," I said. My "big moment" was being driven up in the carriage and waving good-bye. I wasn't worried about it and neither was John. I sat down in my canvas chair while Jennifer Zide, the young makeup woman from San Francisco, redid my lips and powdered me down. I was grateful for the slight delay, as my head felt like a helium balloon.

We rehearsed the drive-up for the camera. Then we did it again for the camera. Then we did it for us, the actors. A little bit of talking, "M.O.S," which is code for "mid-out sound," a traditional humorous expression attributed to the famous director Fritz Lang, calling for a scene "without sound" in his German accent. At least that's the legend. A little bit of waving and nodding and kissing Scarlett good-bye. More blush and lipstick touch-ups. A few words from John: "Slightly more animated, girls. Remember you're all mildly excited here."

Finally we began to shoot. The first shot was okay for us, no good for the cameras: The focus-puller said he thought he could do better. Second try: We actors were a little sluggish, John thought. Third try: We lost the light when the sun hid behind a fluffy cloud. But now it was lunchtime, so the entire company was transported back to the parking lot, where tables and chairs had been set up in a building on the edge of the bay.

I was helped out of my dress and bonnet and went to get a meal tray in my petticoats and shirt. But when I returned to my trailer, I was having trouble breathing. I turned up the air conditioner, but the food was suddenly very unappealing. I drank some water and lay down in the shipshape little bedroom.

Don't Die of Embarrassment

Around two o'clock we were called to get ready. A costume assistant helped me into the dress after I had brushed my teeth and taken some vitamins. Perhaps big doses of E and beta-carotene, along with the daily pill, would make me feel better. When I entered the makeup trailer, Jennifer said, "Barbara, you need more rouge, I think. You're awfully pale." I didn't want to tell her I could barely see her.

Back to the location. Third try: Joanne had some trouble getting out of the carriage, and I dropped my glove into the street. Fourth try: The horse balked a little. He was hot too. Fifth try: Everything worked.

We had very little coverage to do, as John had planned the scene to be our arrival and just one "rehearsal" of Julie Harris coming down the walk to greet her daughter-in-law, Scarlett. We finished at around four in the afternoon, and I was delivered to my very pleasant hotel around five.

CHAPTER 4

Back to the Hotel

I set up my computer and ordered a room-service drink. I was not going to give in to this weakness and become a flu or food-poisoning victim. No, indeed. It was a temporary nonsense. I would work in the room, have my vodka, and phone Jay in New York and the kids in California. Then I would go to the good restaurant in the hotel, get a full night's sleep, run a mile in the morning before my ten o'clock call, and be back to my normal, if slightly thin, self.

But I never got to do any of that, except drink half of the vodka. By seven o'clock I was bleeding profusely. From the rectum. Not a lot of fun. *Very* messy. (Yes, this is extremely plain language we're speaking.) I tried to get to the bed but began to fall down. I leaned against the wall for a minute until the nausea passed. I, who could play three sets of doubles, two of singles, and run miles each day, couldn't stand up without support? Whose white, pasty face peered at me from the dresser mirror? Surely no one I had ever seen before. I held on to consciousness until I fell onto the coverlet and passed out or slept for about an hour. Then I looked in the Yellow Pages and called a doctor who, the ad declared, specialized in colorectal maladies.

A cultivated, slightly removed voice answered. "Atkins here." Oh dear, I had probably interrupted his dinner.

"Sorry to bother you," I said. The room was rocking like a rowboat on a stormy day. "My name is Barbara Barrie, and I'm at the Omni Hotel."

"Yes?"

"I think I'm experiencing a little emergency here."

"What seems to be happening?" The sound of ice tinkled in glass.

"Well, I'm extremely weak, and I can't stop bleeding."

"Bleeding from where, please?"

"The . . . uh . . . the rectum." Embarrassed, I realized that I was loathe to reveal the nature of this illness. How long had I been denying what was going on? And how long *had* anything been going on?

"What have you done so far?" he asked.

I grabbed the headboard to keep the nausea down. "I've stuffed tons of tissues into my panties."

"That's not too specific."

"If I get any more specific, Doctor, they'll arrest me for a lewd phone call."

"Not too funny, Miss Barrie." More ice tinkling. "I really don't have time to waste."

I just hated this guy.

"Is there any way you can help me?" I asked.

"Well, it's quite late now. I'm really not available until the morning."

"Can you give me another name?" I asked. "I don't think I'll make it alone for much longer."

An exasperated sigh. "Okay," he said. "Go to St. Francis Hospital, get them to look at you, and call me after they do a preliminary."

"You don't want to meet me there?"

"No, Miss . . . ah . . ."

"Barrie."

Another sigh. "Yes, Miss Barrie. They're very good at St. Francis, and they'll call me later." The phone, as they say in mystery novels, went "Click!" He was gone.

FADE OUT

CHAPTER 5

Hospital Charleston

St. Francis is a small, private hospital. The emergency waiting room held three people, one with a coughing child in her
lap. I limped up to the desk, asked for instructions, and
expected to fill out the usual nine hundred and fifty docu-
ments while waiting to see someone in a white uniform. But
as the receptionist questioned me, I had to hang on to the
desk. I was not only having trouble locating her face, I also
couldn't hear a thing. I felt as though the blackout was
moments away. Suddenly a hand grasped mine and a voice
said, "Come with me."

A male in a clean white uniform. He took me into a small,
spotless room. Oh joy. A cool, narrow cot. I lay down as this
kind stranger covered me with a sheet.

"Don't I have to sign anything?" I asked. My voice
sounded like that of a three-year-old toddler.

"Not the way you're looking. Tell me what the problem is."

"I'm bleeding . . ."

"Bleeding?" he asked, as he fastened paper to a clipboard.

"Yes, from the . . ." Again I hesitated. I certainly was holding on (an intended pun, for sure) to this information. "From
the . . . rectum."

"Ah," he said, nodding his head and looking wise.

"I can't see very well, and I'm now just reading lips."

"You can't hear?"

"Barely."

"Okay." He wound a blood pressure sleeve around my arm. "Relax. My name is Kent Tretault. We're going to take care of you."

He took my temperature. A middle-aged woman came in to do an EKG, the cold jelly she placed at each pressure point making me jump. After she left with the monitored, squiggly lined paper in her hand, Kent pulled up a leather stool.

"Miss Barrie, have you ever had this kind of bleeding before?"

"Episodes, you know, but never this steadily and for such a long time." (Except that I had had a few bad sieges in London. Too much blood on the white bathroom tiles. Why hadn't I been alarmed then? Or had I?) "Can you stop the bleeding?"

"It already stopped itself. Don't worry," he said, placing a comforting hand on mine. "Have you seen a doctor about this?"

"For years," I said. "Many doctors. They always said it was one thing or another."

"When did this begin?"

"In 1957, I think, but I didn't pay much attention to it."

Kent poured me a glass of water. "Drink this, please, as much as you can. You're very dehydrated."

I propped up on an elbow. The room had stopped turning around, but I felt like an old polo shirt left to dry in the sun. "Thank you," I said, as I gratefully began to sip.

He turned the page on his clipboard. "Family history?"

I averted my eyes. Damn. I knew he'd ask me that. "I'm ashamed to tell you that I'm not sure, but I think we've had a lot of this."

He looked up. "Colorectal cancer?"

"Yes." Finally, I had said it. How long had it been in my subconscious? What the hell was the matter with me?

"Hm-m-m-m-m."

"What does 'hm-m-m-m-m' mean? You don't look happy, Kent," I said.

"You're sixty-two now, Miss Barrie?" He wasn't answering my question.

"Correct."

"Okay." He stood up. "Let me call a really good doctor for you, the best gastroenterologist in Charleston."

"Not Dr. Hideous, the one from the Yellow Pages?" I asked, immediately relieved.

"Definitely not. That guy is . . . uh, well . . . not right for you. Keep drinking the water please." He put another blanket over me and gathered his things. "I'll be back in a minute. Just rest here. You'll be fine."

"Okay." As the door was closing I called, "By the way, why did you take me so quickly?"

"Because you looked very sick. I thought you were going to pass out right there in the entrance."

"I can't thank you enough. You've treated me so well, and I have to finish shooting a TV film tomorrow."

"You what?" He whirled around. "*Scarlett?* You're in *Scarlett?* Oh, of course, you're Barbara Barrie. You're Mrs. Barney Miller. I knew I recognized you! I'm calling Dr. Burns. Oh, wow. This is something. Now relax, I'll be right back."

I lay in the small gleaming room. I knew what this probably was. True, I had been bleeding on and off for years, but in the last year it had become much worse, and I had not gone for a colonoscopy—the thorough examination of the colon—even though my internist had said I must. To call it "in denial" was too mild. How stupid was I? This delay had probably harmed me. So much for a college degree, a thousand years of psychoanalysis, health foods, high fiber, low fat, and forty years of exercise programs. Dumb.

Dr. F. Avery Burns Jr. was everyone's fantasy of a doctor. Tall, soft-spoken, gentle, very Southern. Not Jewish. This was an oddity: I live in New York. Most of the doctors in my life have been Jewish. Rumpled, chicken-fatty, reassuring daddy-substitutes.

He read Kent's report and examined me. A lot of unpleasant anal probing. He kept saying "Sorry" every time I yelped. He asked more questions:

"What were you told, through the years, this bleeding was?"

"I wasn't always bleeding," I protested.

"But when you did . . . ?"

"Oh, internal hemorrhoids, external hemorrhoids, the fissure, tension, you name it."

"When was the first actual diagnosis?"

"In 1958. It was a fissure, and the doctor seemed to think it was coming from stress."

"Why? What was happening?"

"I was doing *The Crucible* every night, off-Broadway, and each day I was rehearsing, also in the city, for Shakespeare repertory at Stratford, Connecticut. I just didn't have much time to sleep, so I thought it would all go away."

"But it got worse?"

"Yes, and my beau at that time found me Dr. Tuchman, who is still my doctor, by the way."

He put down his notes. "Oh, yes, Kent told me you're an actress."

"Trying to be," I answered.

"What did Dr. Tuchman prescribe?"

"A 'white' diet: potatoes, ice cream, cream of wheat—that kind of thing. And a little success. He said that in a month, once we opened at Stratford—my main role was Hermia in *A Midsummer Night's Dream*—I would relax."

Dr. Burns smiled. "And were you successful?"

I could hardly speak; the memories of that green summer suddenly invaded in an almost physical way. It had been one of the most extraordinary experiences of my life, playing great classics in the beautiful theater, driving home each night in my snub-nosed secondhand Studebaker convertible as the moon sent silver dust, like Puck's, over the Housatonic River.

"Yes," I finally said. "And the fissure went away."

"Miss Barrie," he said quietly, "I want you to stay in the hospital tonight, and we'll do a colonoscopy tomorrow."

I sat up quickly. Two hammers seemed to hit my head, one on each side, but I said, "I just can't do that." I was panicking. "I've got to shoot tomorrow."

"Shoot? What do you mean, 'shoot'?"

"I'm making a film here . . . *Scarlett.*"

"What is that?"

"A mini-series we're doing in Charleston for CBS."

"You can't be serious."

"Dr. Burns, it's my last day. My acting partner is having trouble with her knee. I've got to be there to help her."

"Her knee?"

"Yes, I can't explain. She's my age, she won't get them fixed. Please let me finish, then I can go back to New York and get all the rest of the tests done there."

He gazed at me. "I see." The room was silent. I had visions of ruining the film, of being considered a quitter, of harming John Erman's reputation, of failing in my responsibility. Dying never occurred to me.

He crossed his arms. After another long pause he said, "Suppose we do this. You stay here tonight. We'll do the test in the morning. We have to look in there and see what's going on. Then, if you can, we'll send you back to work."

Suddenly exhausted, I lay back down. "Thank you very much. Would you mind calling my doctor in New York?"

"Good idea. Dr. Tuchman, you mean. Yes, give me his number, please."

FADE OUT.

FADE IN

APRIL 7, 1994
ST. FRANCIS HOSPITAL, 1:15 A.M.

That night I drank a gallon of something called "Golytely." Yes, it means exactly what it says. Except you don't go lightly.

You go suddenly and then constantly, and it keeps you up for hours. At least I had a fascinating book, *Wild Swans* by Jung Chang, about life during the cultural revolution in China, so I had reading material in the bathroom, out of the bathroom, sitting in the chair, brushing my teeth, drinking the god-damned Golytely. Compared to the tribulations of families under Mao, my problems were paltry.

What would happen to me now? If this was really cancer, how far had it spread? How much time did I have to live? Could the tumor, for surely it was a tumor, possibly be benign?

Between trips to the bathroom, I began to doze and dream in fragments, like pieces of a Cézanne painting, floating in a color wash, greeny-orange, then beige, a cottage, a tree, brown-gold now, divided into sections like his Aix farm fields.

Greenwich Village about forty years ago, my three room-mates and I lived in the old Astor mansion across from the Public Theater on Lafayette Street, keeping house, dividing the grocery bills, playing the piano, looking for theater work, holding down "day jobs," going to voice lessons, ballet and acting classes.

Each girl paid twenty-five dollars a month—one hundred dollars for a two-thousand-square-foot apartment. Our living room had been the Astor ballroom, complete with raised platform for the long-ago orchestras, where men in tails and women in extravagant ball gowns waltzed around the palm-filled room.

Oh yes, one night, I remember that night . . . it was my turn to wash the dishes, Charlotte was to dry. As I handed a plate to her, I felt a pain in my belly and an urgent need to go to the bathroom. The sensation was becoming familiar: It had started occurring after every meal.

"Charlotte, I have to take a bathroom break."

"Barbara, you always do that when you have to do the dishes." She was tall, funny, gorgeous, at that time playing in *Gypsy* on Broadway.

"I know, that's true. But I just have to."

"Just finish the washing, and I'll clean up the kitchen," said Jo, another of the roommates, who was clearing the table. "I've got a jazz class, but not for an hour."

"Okay, good deal." I didn't want to be a crybaby. My dignity was at stake. And the pain got worse. When I had done the last glass, I rushed to the bathroom. But it was too late. I was unsuccessful. I felt my stomach close and bloat.

New fragments of memory now. I remember doubling over, feeling sick, the old, hexagonal bathroom tiles blending black lines into a mottled design. Had I lost control of my own body by not listening to it? Why hadn't I just left the kitchen? Why was I so afraid to speak up? Was I so fearful of being disliked? I was wildly uncomfortable, and I didn't know how to fix it. If I straightened up, the cramps became impossible, but I was getting light-headed in that bent-over position.

Now, under this blanket in Charleston, I moved my head from side to side. I saw myself at twenty-four, puzzled and handicapped somehow in the weeks and months that followed that long-ago night. Not seeking help. Gulping different kinds of laxatives. Worried that my secret might be serious. Had that been the beginning of the journey to this point?

The Golytely was almost finished. As dawn arrived, Kent, his shift over, came in to say good night. "Good luck, Miss Barrie. If you have any problems at all, here's the emergency room number, and here's my home phone. My wife, Darla, is a nurse too. I've told everyone here to look out for you."

How's that for sensitive care in a small South Carolina hospital? Thank God for "Barney Miller" and for goodhearted souls in white uniforms like Kent Tretault.

FADE OUT

FADE IN

S<small>T</small>. F<small>RANCIS</small> H<small>OSPITAL</small>, 8:00 <small>A.M.</small>

"What kind of music do you like, Miss Barrie?"

We were in an immaculate room. This one with a mysterious, blinking machine and a first-rate stereo system. I was still reading *Wild Swans*. Anything to pretend I was a calm, educated, swell person.

"Do you have any Beethoven?"

"You bet." The starched nurses smiled, patted my shoulders, smoothed my hair, and turned on the tape. Utterly glorious. I was going to be just dandy.

Dr. Burns entered. "Your doctor said that if this is a tumor, it's only in the rectum. He may be right because I could feel it with my finger last night."

"What does that mean?"

"That we won't do a full colonoscopy, even though I believe we should. We might find something else. He doesn't want you to have a transfusion. I told him that the blood supply in Charleston is much cleaner than in New York . . ."

"Are we speaking of AIDS?"

"Exactly. You don't absolutely have to have a transfusion, although it would make you feel much better—you've lost a lot of blood—but the colonoscopy is up to you."

"I'd rather not. Won't I be dopey?"

"No. We'll give you a little Valium now, and you'll be fine in less than an hour."

"I just can't. Elizabeth Wilson and I have two tough scenes together. I can't show up weaving around like a drunk."

He laughed. "Okay, we'll give you the shot, and we'll just do a sigmoidoscopy. It'll all be over in fifteen minutes. Please turn on your right side."

Oh no. They were really going to send this little camera up my behind. Whatever they were going to find would be the real truth, the terrible truth that I had known, I think, for many months. Clutching *Wild Swans,* I drifted off to the second movement of Beethoven's Piano Concerto No. 3.

About eleven minutes later I woke up. It had been painless. If I had known this, I would have had the test years before. Dumb, dumb, *dumb.* Soon Dr. Burns handed me the pictures he had taken. There, amid regular-looking red tissue, was an ugly-looking, white, miniature volcano. Like the ones you see in children's books of dinosaurs and other prehistoric phenomena. I was a walking Jurassic landscape, waiting to explode.

"What do you think, Dr. Burns?"

"I'm not certain." He was avoiding my gaze, and we both knew it. "You'd have to have a biopsy before we'd be sure of anything."

We shook hands. "Try to take it easy today, and please keep me informed when you get back to New York."

"I will," I said.

CHAPTER 6

Last Day of Shooting

I dressed quickly and signed release papers. I blessed the Screen Actors Guild for the best health plan in any working person's life.

At eight-thirty that morning I took a cab to the set, was stuffed into the corset, two petticoats, ankle boots, and a two-piece, majestically embroidered silk dress.

Elizabeth Wilson and I, seated in our chairs, watched our stand-ins rehearse the carriage ride to the bottom of the steps, climb out, and ascend the fifty steps. It looked simple. No dialogue, just physical activity. A cinch.

"Where were you last night, Barbara, dear?" she asked, as we fanned ourselves in the heat. "Do you know that when I couldn't reach you by eleven o'clock, I had the hotel unlock your room?"

"You're kidding."

"Indeed, I'm not. I could tell you hadn't been feeling well, and I was so worried. Especially when you didn't call me at dinnertime. I went in with the security people, but we couldn't find any clues, so I thought maybe you had a secret meeting somewhere, and perhaps I should just keep quiet."

"Oh, Liz, you are such a romantic! I'm sixty-two years old."

"Well, darling, what difference does that make?"

I thought I'd better tell the truth. "Liz, please don't say anything, but I was pretty sick and went to the hospital, and they kept me overnight for tests."

"Oh my God, what kinds of tests?"

"I can't go into detail now. We mustn't worry John, but I'll tell you everything tonight."

Our stand-ins rehearsed the scene for about an hour. When the camera operator felt he had the shot perfectly planned, we took our places. The vehicle came into view and stopped. On the mark, perfect. We started to get out. My huge skirt covered the little iron steps of the carriage, and I couldn't see where to put my feet. Liz, because of her bad knee, had a terrible time getting down to the pavement.

"Cut!"

John walked over. "It's difficult, hmm?"

I felt humiliated. "Well, yes, John. Our stand-ins had blue jeans and sneakers on. It's not the same." I had to blame someone.

"Oh, I see," he said. "Okay, just try again, and just lift up the skirts . . ."

"Higher than we think we should," I added.

"Exactly." He stepped behind the camera, and again we took our places. "Roll. *Action!*" he called.

This time we managed not to trip and started up the stairs. Liz was protecting her knee, and I, sleepless, felt that my chest was rubbing against my backbone. I was like a toy figure on a stick—the kind whose arms and legs move by pulling down the string. I was walking, but orange polkadots were dancing in front of my eyes, and every breath was an achievement.

At the top of the stairs, we stopped. We had made it. Elizabeth and I grinned at each other. We heard a dismayed, "Cut!"

John Erman dashed up the steps. "Girls, girls, I'm going to make you do it over."

"Oh, John, why?" we wailed, almost in unison.

"We thought we were wonderful," I said.

"Girls, I don't know what movie you're playing in, but it's not this one."

"Oh, John, tell us," I pleaded, as the prop people brought our canvas chairs. Thankfully, we sank down. A young intern brought us water, which we practically threw into our mouths. It was terrifyingly hot.

John squatted down at our side. "Do you remember the scene we did two days ago in the railroad station? You were both fluttering and gesticulating and waving the tickets around? Scarlett walked between you?"

"Of course," we replied. We had loved that scene. It had been such fun whizzing the whole length of the "station" (it was really the Federal Building of Charleston). We had improvised our dialogue, changing it every time we had done another "take."

"Well, this scene precedes that. We've already seen you animated and looking forward to the train trip. Today you are like two old ladies laboring up these steps . . ."

"We *are* two old ladies," we protested.

"No," he laughed, "you are two wonderful actresses, and I want you to act. Let's have a little life here. Remember, we next see you flying through the entrance of the railroad station. Now let's try again."

He offered his hand to Liz, who winced as she rose from her chair. "Darling, is your knee hurting?"

"A little, John dear, but honestly it's a twinge, nothing at all. I'm just being foolish."

Gathering our crinolines, we walked to the horse and carriage.

The cinematographer, Tony Imi, joined us. "Why don't we lose the pull-up, John, and just catch the ladies as they start up the steps?" I was so dizzy that I was clutching the buggy wheel to keep from pitching forward into the fake gravel.

"Good idea," said John.

Once more Jennifer Zide patted my damp face with a sponge. Marit Allen adjusted my bonnet. The temperature was now close to 90 degrees, but in our finery it felt like 110. I wasn't sure I was going to be able to climb those steps one more time. The sun was blinding when John said, "Babs, you okay? You look a little peaked."

"I'm okay, thanks," I said.

The last take was the winner. Elizabeth and I, talking to each other, laughing, bounded up the fifty steps. Well, "bounded," is not quite the right word, but we did get up there as the two fussy women we were supposed to be playing.

"Print!" John called and ran up to us. "Girls, girls, you were just fabulous. Thank you. That was perfect."

And perspiring, relieved, and seriously lacking blood, I was "wrapped" from *Scarlett.*

CHAPTER 7

First Visit to Dr. Eng

My internist had made an appointment for me with a specialist in colon and rectal surgery the day after I came home from Charleston. At four o'clock, April 12, at New York University Medical Center, I was seated across the desk from young, cheerful Dr. Eng. I gave him the test pictures from Charleston. The little volcano. Impassively, he studied it.

He asked me the usual questions: family history, symptoms, all the questions I had been asked in Charleston, the same ones that would be repeated throughout my journey with this disease.

None of it seemed at all mysterious to him. Before he took me into the examination room, I was sure he knew exactly what I had and exactly what he was going to have to do.

"Let's go have a look."

"It's cancerous, isn't it?"

"I don't know until I examine you and until I have a biopsy report."

"But it looks awful in the picture."

"But these are not my pictures." His self-assurance was overwhelming. Maybe I'd better just keep still. "I won't make a diagnosis until I have my own results."

"Oh, of course."

"Now let Charlotte take you into the other room."

Again a nurse. Again the crinkly paper sheet, the antiseptic light. Once more the humiliating, awkward exam. Naked from the waist down, I lay on my side like a curled-up fetus. This absolute stranger had his finger up my rectum, and he was very, very quiet. The only sound was my grunting and puffing against the pain.

I could only see the nurse's face, but as Dr. Eng removed the biopsy sample, she looked slightly, just slightly, shocked. As he straightened up, they glanced at each other, their conclusions hanging in the air between them like a string of tiny Christmas lights.

"Come back in a week when the tests are ready," he said, taking off the latex gloves.

"It's what I thought, isn't it?"

Measuring his words carefully, he said, "It may be, but we'll have to get the results."

He had seen too many tumors. I knew he was not telling the truth, and he knew I knew it.

"What if it's really cancer?" I asked.

"Let's wait for a while, shall we?"

"I'll have to wear a pouch, won't I? You'll have to do a colostomy."

"Miss Barrie, don't jump to conclusions, please."

That did it. I collapsed into his arms, and he patted me. "You'll be just fine." He was calm. Obviously many patients collapsed into his arms, but I hadn't wanted to be one of them. I had wanted to be Greer Garson as Mrs. Miniver, or Barbara Stanwyck, bravely lifting her chin as Lolly left her for the "swell life." A staunch, steady person who could weather any crisis. Forget it. I was Barbara, drenching the white coat of Dr. Eng.

I boarded the First Avenue bus in a numb fog. Why had I meticulously taken care of every other aspect of my health and ignored the one area of my body that had always been a problem?

What had I been thinking? That if I found out the truth, then I might be an invalid, I might die, that I'd be like . . . who was it . . . someone in my family, maybe two someones, who had had something wrong with their colons, or was it the rectum, or no . . . maybe the stomach?

For many years I had had an "irritable bowel," diagnosed four months after that awful night in Greenwich Village. When they were little, Jane and Aaron complained that I spent more time in the bathroom than I did with them. I did get a fabulous amount of reading done: *The New Yorker*, cover to cover; *The Saturday Review of Literature*; *Gourmet Magazine* (from which no recipes were ever tried); and bulletins from the children's schools. Besides, it was my private time: no phones, no "Mommy!," no household dilemmas. It was just lovely.

This last year I knew the bleeding had increased, but I had let it go. When I had lost over ten pounds in a short time, I'd convinced myself that it was the result of not eating fat and exercising more. Besides, I looked great in my clothes. Who would want to disturb that?

As I transferred to the crosstown bus on 72nd Street, I admitted to myself that I almost surely had cancer. In 1940 we had moved from the bayside tourist court to a tract house in the middle of a former cotton field in Corpus Christi. My father began to make a little money. I had my own room with a white bed and a ruffled dressing table. My mother had stopped complaining about her life.

Every night I had rolled up my hair in socks, and in the mornings I had put on saddle shoes and broomstick skirts with rickrack along the hems. I had learned to drive a car at fifteen. I had ridden a skittery horse named Victory during World War II, played tennis in the public parks, picnicked with my friends on the beach at Padre Island.

I had been in love all through high school with a freckle-faced football player named Edwin Meisenheimer. He had been my confidant, my best friend. I had been chums with the same eccentric, wonderful girls since the fourth grade. We had all gone to "air-cooled" movies downtown on Saturday nights and to the Friday night "Twixteen" dances at the Episcopal church, where we had jitterbugged and slow-danced and afterward ate cheeseburgers with mayonnaise and onions at Pick's Drive Inn.

How could I have gotten cancer?

CHAPTER 8

Second Visit
to Dr. Eng

APRIL 19, 1994

Today I would hear the results of the biopsy, although I
already knew what they would be. During the last week, Jay
and I had given a small, impromptu dinner party and had
seen a play on Broadway. I'd done three loads of laundry,
gone to the gym, and bought a new pair of suede pumps (to
wear in the hospital?). I purchased my subway tokens and
my lunch-counter salads and read the *New York Times* as
though nothing were hanging in the balance. I had wrapped
myself in a cocoon of calm: What else could I do?

My friend Carol Perlberger had come to see the new apartment. Carol had been an art major in college, and she has a
fabulous eye for architecture and detail and a wealth of ideas
about the use of space.

Dust and plaster covered everything, and the rat-tat of the
hammers was contrasted by large tools being dropped, the
chatter of five different Chinese dialects being spoken by
the skilled workmen, and the phone ringing as if our house
were the box office of the latest Broadway smash hit.

Carol and I took our iced tea and sat on the bed in the bedroom amid the packing cases, the rolled-up rugs, and the
paintings stacked against the freshly painted walls.

"You've done a wonderful job, Barbara. I have to admit it—you've thought of everything."

"Thanks," I said. "Your opinion is important to me."

There were two scenarios being played: one was talk of the apartment, of our children, our husbands, of a law case being played on Court TV, the latest to-do in the Clinton administration. The other was the dialogue in my head:

"Carol, guess what? I have cancer. It's pretty bad, I think. A tumor is eating its way through my body, and I will probably have to wear a plastic bag for the rest of my life. If I live. If I don't die from the operation. If I get rid of this cancer, and another doesn't appear later on."

I didn't say anything. And I was still not ready to disclose anything to anyone other than Jay. I didn't want to be a victim. I didn't want to be my mother after my father died— lying in a darkened room every afternoon with a cold cloth on her head, crying and asking me to bring her water or aspirin or iced coffee. I wanted to be an alive person, not afraid, not cowed by this illness.

Dr. Eng walked briskly into the office, a biopsy report in his hand. He sat down at his desk and folded his hands.

"Well, Miss Barrie," he said softly, "it's a carcinoma of the rectum, and it's very low . . ."

"So you won't be able to just stitch me up."

"Right, it'll be a colostomy."

Boom. Just like that. My heart doubled over inside, and my body seemed to melt like a Dalí clock over the leather chair.

"The bright side is that these low tumors can be treated successfully much of the time. The prognosis is better, believe it or not, than if the tumor was high in the colon."

I noticed the pictures of his wife and children on the wall behind him. A shiny-haired, grinning boy and a doll-like little girl. His wife, slight and charming. Dr. Eng had a life. He didn't have to worry about a tumor. What luck he had, and how jealous I was.

"Will I have to have radiation and chemotherapy?"

"It depends on how far this has developed. We have to wait until we really get a look."

"When do you want to do this operation?" I was suddenly very businesslike, organized.

"We'll admit you tomorrow."

"What? Tomorrow? Are you serious?" Now I was not at all calm or organized.

"I am serious. Come in the morning, and Friday we'll do the procedure. My assistant will get all the details and make the necessary arrangements."

He rose from his chair and extended his hand. "Don't worry about anything. We'll take good care of you."

And he was gone. I sat there wrapped in a strange, terrifying paralysis. Well, this was it. The little volcano was really cancer. I would probably have to have radiation and chemotherapy, and I would have to wear the bag—the dreaded nightmare of anybody with a colon problem.

Dr. Eng's assistant, tall, perfectly groomed, whisked through the door and sat in the doctor's chair. She wore a chignon and had the air of the school principal who has called you in for bad behavior in your fifth-grade history class.

"What kind of insurance do you have, Miss Barrie?"

"Uh . . . Screen Actors Guild—Travelers." My mouth was dry. I felt as if I were in someone else's dream.

"Who will accompany you to the hospital?"

"My husband, I guess."

"Please be at the admitting office at . . ."

I fell slightly apart. Not completely. I didn't want this cold person to think I wasn't in control, but the abrupt reality of what lay ahead was closing my throat and making my hands shake.

"What's wrong, Miss Barrie?" Was she nuts?

"Well, this is . . . I mean now that I'm really facing this, it's . . ." Damn! Here came the tears again. I reached for a tissue in my bag, but none was there.

Not moving at all, she looked at me with the principal's

eyes. And she didn't say a word. We looked at each other silently for what seemed three weeks.

"Do you have a tissue, Miss . . . what is your name, please?"

"Mrs. Kucynski." She reached into a drawer and handed me a small box.

"Don't you think, Mrs. Kucynski, that this is a common reaction?"

"Yes, it's quite common."

"Well . . . why are you so . . ." I couldn't continue. She wasn't going to offer any comfort or wisdom at all.

"Please check in tomorrow at eight o'clock. You'll be in the hospital approximately twelve days, until we're sure everything is functioning properly. Now if you'll just fill out this paper, I'll make all the appointments."

She left the room, and Dr. Eng returned.

"Everything okay, Miss Barrie?"

"I guess so." My head seemed to be taking the shape of a blowfish—huge, puffed-out. "But I'm quite apprehensive."

"Of course you are. Who wouldn't be? But you'll do just fine." At last an understanding word.

"What exactly happens in this operation?" I asked.

"I'll remove the tumor and the rectum." Inside I quietly fell apart again, but I just stared at him. "As we now know, the tumor is too low to save the rectum."

How does one live without a rectum? "Oh God." His children gazed sweetly from the pictures. "What else?"

"Then we redirect the bowel and make a new opening on the left side of your belly. The opening is called a 'stoma.'"

What a brutal word. Like "stone" or "stomp." Or a combination of both. "That's where the bag goes?" I asked, still recoiling from the word itself.

"Yes. It will be a small opening, like a rosebud really."

A rosebud? I almost threw up.

"Yes, I don't like it to be larger than that, and we have people here who will teach you all about handling it, how to irrigate your body every day." Someone who would assist me with my bodily excretions? It seemed unreal and dreadful.

"I'll operate about noon."

"I see."

"And then I leave for my vacation."

"Your what?" Now it wasn't a dream, it was a nightmare. No, it was a satire.

"My vacation."

"How long will you be gone?"

"Two weeks."

"You're going to operate and then leave?"

"Oh, yes. All the doctors in my department are excellent. I guarantee if there's any problem at all, and I don't expect there to be, the doctors here all do the same procedure; you'll be very safe."

"Could I think about this?"

"Of course." He leaned forward. "Except that I won't be here after Friday."

"Um-m-m." I could barely nod my head.

"If you like, you can wait until I get back."

"Two weeks?"

"It won't make much difference."

"Why not?"

"These tumors grow very slowly." He smiled strangely. The subtext was, "You've let this go so long that more time will neither help nor harm you." At least, in my paranoia, that's what I thought he was inferring.

"Well, give me a day to consider everything," I said, clutching the now-wadded tissue.

"Of course, but I urge you to go ahead with the procedure."

"Thank you." We shook hands. "You know, Dr. Eng, I would prefer to have you here during the recovery."

"Miss Barrie, I understand. But I guarantee that we will do a successful operation. This is what I do. I know how to do it, and you'll be in capable hands."

I was reeling by this time. What if something went wrong,

and the doctor was snorkeling somewhere in the Pacific? What if the cancer had spread so far that there was nothing they could do? What if they found it in my liver, and they had to take a piece of that too? I wanted Dr. Eng's advice, not an intern's or a resident's.

Call me childish, call me selfish, call me panicked. I was all of those things, and in addition, I was totally bewildered and right now very, very angry.

I rose and grabbed my purse. "May I call you later today or tomorrow?"

"Of course."

I walked out past the secretaries, past Mrs. Kucynski, who once again just stared at me. I didn't say good-bye.

CHAPTER 9

The Gottliebs

That night I called two of our closest friends, Elisabeth Scharlatt, an editor, and Paul Gottlieb, the head of an art publishing firm. They had been married only a few years, a second marriage for each, and they were like the fizz on the top of a champagne glass.

Elisabeth recently had had a benign tumor removed from her colon. ("Paul married me and two seconds later had to take care of me!") They both had spoken with awe about her surgeon at Columbia Presbyterian Hospital.

"If the guy's going to operate and leave for two weeks . . . I mean, my God, you can't let him do it. I don't care if he's brilliant, you simply can't do it," Paul sputtered. I was certain that steam was coming from his nostrils, and his large, handsome face would be apoplectically magenta. He takes friendship very seriously.

"Barbara, this is me," Elisabeth said. "I'm on the other phone. You must see Dr. Kelly. He's remarkable."

"Elisabeth," Jay interrupted, "our internist says this guy at NYU is the best surgeon in the city for a colostomy. Maybe she should go ahead and do it now, not delay."

"But Jay," Paul said, "it's good to have a second opinion. What if there's a better way to do the operation? What if Kelly could make it less severe? That's a huge procedure. You have to find out more."

"Barbara, it's me, Elisabeth," she said breathlessly.

"Yes, Elisabeth. I know."

"Shall we call him first?" she asked. "Do you want us to go with you? What can we do?"

"Well, would you mind calling him and paving the way for me?" I asked. I hated the idea of having to go over this whole thing again with another doctor, but at this point I really wanted another opinion. Maybe I could avoid the colostomy.

"We'll call him right away," said Paul. "I'll tell him how adorable you are. Now just rest easy. Everything will be fine. Don't worry." His breathing was slowing down to a quiet roar.

"Barbara, it's me, Elisabeth."

I smiled. "Yes, I know, Elisabeth."

"We love you. And we'll call you as soon as we talk to Dr. Kelly. Please don't worry. We don't want you to do anything hasty."

"Okay, I won't."

"Love you, darling," said Paul. "Jay, you okay?"

"Just fine, thanks." But I could hear a tenseness, a weariness in Jay's voice.

"Pour yourselves a big drink and look at your view," said Elisabeth. "We'll call you tomorrow."

"What are you thinking, Jay?" I asked as we met in the kitchen. I wanted him to have a firm opinion. I longed to have some of the responsibility taken away from me.

"I think it's the most astounding coincidence that Elisabeth has just had the operation you need, except that yours, of course, is in the rectum, and hers was in the colon."

I took some apples from the refrigerator. "But how do you feel? What do you think should be my next step?"

He poured red wine into two glasses. "I feel huge relief. The fact that our dearest friends can recommend someone so highly is encouraging, don't you think?"

"Yes, I do." We moved back into the living room. It was almost time for the eleven o'clock news. "So should I see this other guy?"

"Barbara, it's a hard decision, but I definitely want you to make the appointment. Then we'll decide. If you're so uncomfortable with Dr. Eng's being gone after the operation, you've probably got to choose someone else."

Jay turned on the television, and we settled into the pillows. "Okay, it looks, at least, as if I'll have a choice."

I called Dr. Eng's office and canceled the operation, at least for now. Mrs. Cold Heart only said, "Very well. I'll tell the doctor."

I called Marcel Tuchman. "You're making a mistake, Barbara. He's really the best, and you should have this done immediately."

"But Marcel, he's going on vacation. Should I be operated on by someone who's going to be unavailable?"

"I'll be there, Barbara, and Dr. Kahn will be there. It's the best hospital in the city, and that's where you should be."

I stopped cold. I had forgotten, in the melee of this cancer business, Dr. Kahn, the cardiologist. Two years before I had had a heart "episode," which had resulted in an angiogram and an angioplasty. "If I have a heart attack on the table, Marcel," I said, "I guess the cancer won't matter."

"You're not going to have a heart attack, my dear, and the cancer will be cured. The prognosis for this is excellent." His musical Polish accent almost lulled me into saying, "Yes." After forty years I trusted him completely, even though I didn't always do what he said. Ah, portent of things to come.

"I'm so confused, Marcel."

"The sooner this is done, the better."

I had a feeling he was right, and probably I was finding a way to put off the whole thing. If I postponed it, pretended it didn't exist, maybe it would go away or they'd find that it was a little cyst they had misdiagnosed. Dr. Eng, on the first visit, had cauterized the tumor. Since then I had had much less pain, no blood, and no difficulty in the bathroom.

Barbara Barrie

Two days later Dr. Kelly, at Columbia Presbyterian Hospital, had his finger in the usual place. I met him at eleven o'clock and by eleven-twenty I was lying on my side, naked from the waist down, and he was probing my insides. I was almost getting used to all this, but it was still a shock to be so exposed, so vulnerable with something growing within me that could be doing its harm even as I spoke to this stranger.

He sat down on the little stool. The one where you always put your handbag and the nurse glares at you, and you take it off.

His face was pensive as he smoothed his glossy hair away from his forehead.

"Well, the tumor is low. I can feel it, but maybe we can hitch it up so that you don't have to lose the rectum."

"Oh, that would be a blessing."

"Don't get your hopes up, Miss Barrie, but it's worth a try. At least we should take some pictures and investigate the other possibilities."

Could there be another way? Could this doctor save me from a colostomy?

"Have you had a sonogram or a CAT scan?" he asked.

Why hadn't Dr. Eng ordered a sonogram? Was he going to do it when I entered the hospital? "No. I had a lower examination . . . what do you call that?"

"A sigmoidoscopy. You've had those before, right?"

"Yes, but . . ." I didn't want to tell him that, before Charleston, I hadn't had one in over a year.

"But you neglected this for a while."

Caught. "How did you know?" I asked.

"Because this tumor is really there. You must have known that it was." Looking down at his notes, he was trying to be casual, but I was totally frightened.

"I think I just didn't want to admit it," I said, "for the usual reasons. 'Denial' is my middle name, I guess."

"Yes, well, that happens. Do you have the picture from Charleston?"

I drew the little volcano from my purse. He frowned. Bad sign. "What were you doing in Charleston?"

"Making a mini-series for CBS."

"What do you mean?" he asked, as if I had been speaking from another planet.

"I was acting in a mini-series called *Scarlett*."

"You're an actress?" He seemed to be looking for my space uniform and pointed ears.

"Ummmm."

"Well, uh . . ." It was the first moment since our meeting had begun that he seemed genuinely insecure. "Why don't you get dressed, come into the other room, and we'll talk some more?"

On the wall of his office was a laminated page from *New York* magazine that announced "The One Hundred Best Doctors in Manhattan." I deduced that he must be one of them. And why not? He was thoughtful, attractive; and the Gottliebs had had nothing but praise for him.

"I suggest that we make appointments for the CAT scan and the sonogram right away," he said, looking at his notes. "Then we'll have more information. Let my secretary make the appointments for you, and I'll see you in a week or so."

God, another week, another delay.

Jay and I walked thoughtfully to the parking lot. We backed the car out onto the street without speaking to each other. I was exhausted from self-preoccupation and fell asleep immediately as Jay headed for Fire Island.

Finally on the Grand Central Parkway, as we were passing La Guardia Airport, I sighed heavily and straightened up.

"You really had quite a nap," Jay said, relieved, I think, that I was coming back to life.

"Mm-m-m." I reached for some Life Savers in the glove compartment.

"What did Dr. Kelly say?" he asked, holding out his hand for a mint.

"Well, he offered a little hope. He wants to do more tests. If he can find something to attach my gut to, he may not have to do a colostomy."

"Wouldn't that be great?"

"It's something to cling to, Jay, but I have my doubts." Traffic had stalled now, and we both rolled down our windows.

"Why? You always write such a doom-and-gloom scenario, Barbara."

"Jay, the tumor's too low. Everyone can feel it. I have a confession. I stuck my finger in there. I can feel it too."

"Honestly? You're a brave soul."

"I just wanted to see or feel, as the case may be, what everyone is talking about."

"So what do you think you want to do?" Sirens were coming up behind us. "There must be an accident ahead," he said.

"I don't know what I'm really thinking," I said. "I'm sure I'm just avoiding a decision. Dr. Kelly could probably operate in less than a week."

"But honey, Dr. Eng said that one or two weeks wouldn't make any difference. You could wait until he comes back."

"Yes, but he doesn't have this goddamned thing growing inside of him." An ambulance was struggling to get through the two lanes of traffic. Jay pulled slightly to the left. "I have to do something quickly, don't I?"

"Within a reasonable time, I think. When are we going to tell the kids?" Our children, who were in California writing as a comedy team for television, were working the usual eighteen hours a day on a situation comedy that would premiere in the fall.

"Oh, Jay, not until we know all the details. Why say anything until we have more knowledge?" I put my arm around his shoulder. "They have to be funny, they have to write comedy. This kind of news is all they need right now."

"Barbara, they are big people, all grown up." His face became almost expressionless, as it always did when we had this kind of conversation about the children. "They can take it."

A brick wall fell around my heart. This was not in the plan: not to be the mommy, the strong friend to Jane and Aaron, the woman who could do anything, who never got sick, had indomitable energy, enthusiasm, always available, healthy, cheery, adventuresome Mommy.

But all I said was, "Can we talk about it later?"

"Barbara, they are going to be angry, offended, if you leave them out of this."

"No, they won't," I answered, my voice strident. "Why should I burden them with something they can do nothing about?"

"That's overprotective behavior. You've always been that way, and it's never done them any good."

"Jay, please. This is too hard a decision."

"Okay, but you make me so angry. Your thinking is all wrong."

The trees, newly budding, washed by the windows of the car. We were going to spend a weekend on our beloved Fire Island. But how many weekends would I have left there? Even if I recovered, I might be wearing a plastic bag under my bathing suit and under my tennis clothes, if I ever played again. Would people be able to tell? Would I care if people could tell? How long would there be residual pain?

I napped again. I couldn't seem to stay awake. I had always slept in the car, but this day descended like a gray veil, oppressive, without color, dulling my energy.

When I awoke again I said, "Jay, I keep thinking about the quality of my life: Is it worth it, to go through all these tests and pain and the operation? I'm going to die sometime . . ."

"Gloom and doom. Gloom and doom. We're all going to die sometime, honey. Look at your mother, she's ninety-five and . . ." His voice trailed away.

"And still impossible," I said.

"The Killer Bee," he added.

"Well, I might die just a little sooner than expected, that's all. Do I want to spend the time left in hospitals, under radiation machines, and having poison pumped into my body? Because that's what will probably happen. I think I'd rather just be made comfortable."

"Barb, you're talking rubbish. You don't even have Dr. Kelly's final opinion yet. He said he may be able to avoid the colostomy."

"True, but it looks bleak." As we inched forward, we could see flashing lights in the distance.

"Think about it until Monday. Things will sort themselves out once you throw yourself into the ocean. You know how you love that."

"Playing some good tennis would help too, Jay."

"We could make a little love," he said. "How about that?"

"A perfect suggestion," I answered, although at that moment it seemed low on the list. I kissed his cheek. I couldn't believe his sensitivity and flexibility. Yet it would be almost two years before I would find out what he had really been feeling.

How could he love me? It's a frightful drag to have to worry about a sick person, to have the pall of a disease hanging over all the hours of a couple's lives. And I was a very bossy, overenergized person. And I yelled at him about his snoring and his compulsive saving of magazines and newspapers and his workaholic habits.

"Do you want to go over to Fair Harbor for dinner tonight, Barb?" he said as we finally drew past the accident, a minor one it seemed, involving only one car and a fence. "The usual inexplicable delay caused by a 'gaper-block,'" Jay said explosively. "Why in hell does the traffic always have to stop dead like this?"

"The eternal mystery of the Northern State Parkway," I said as I reached into my purse for the grocery list. "Did you pick up vodka?"

"Yes, two bottles."

"What kind?"

"Oblivion vodka, Barbara. I don't know, Fleischman's, I think."

I punched his arm. "I *hate* Fleischman's! You got it on sale somewhere."

"Of course. Have I ever resisted a bargain?"

"You're a bum. I want Absolut."

"What can I say? I bought the other kind. Now let's talk about tonight. Are you going to tell any of our friends about this?"

"I don't think so. I can't seem to let go of it yet. I still think someone will call and say, 'Miss Barrie, there has been a terrible error, the tests were wacky. You're okay.'"

"You know, you can tell people you have cancer," he said, "and they'll commiserate and cluck their tongues and forget all about it. I hate to tell you, but they won't really care. Oh, I mean, they'll care, but only for a minute or two."

"You're right," I said. "Life goes on, dum-de-dum-dum."

"So telling or not telling is not that big a deal," he said. "Except for the children. That's something you have to do, or you're going to make a big mistake."

Jay put in a tape. We turned up the volume. The car flooded with music. Emanuel Ax playing Chopin's First Piano Concerto.

After a while in the still-slow-moving traffic, I said, "Did you really buy Fleischman's?"

"Barbara, you're going to love it."

We drove on for another few miles. Then he said, "As for telling or not telling people, that's completely up to you. You're the author of this screenplay."

"Thanks," I said, and began to drift away again. It was a relief to turn off my brain, not to feel my tongue, dry from distress, clinging disgustingly against my teeth, not to be opening and closing my mouth all the time like Charlie McCarthy sitting on Edgar Bergen's knee, waving his head from side to side and rolling his eyes.

CHAPTER 10

The CAT Scan

APRIL 25, 1994
COLUMBIA PRESBYTERIAN HOSPITAL

The CAT scan was not at all what I expected. First of all, it takes a long time. I lay on a moving platform, my arms stretched out behind my head. Slipping through a tunnel-like machine, I felt as if I were slowly being drawn over a long, old-fashioned washboard. Slight bump. Pause. Slight bump. Pause. Repeated about sixty times while the scanner is taking a thorough look at the hidden places of the body. It's painless, but I felt like a pile of laundry being subjected to an endless, hard scrub.

My thoughts were adrift, blending like the colored dots in a Seurat painting—gold, blue, red. What would the machine find? Did I remember to start defrosting the chicken for tomorrow's dinner? Would my numb arms ever come down again? Why was I so calm? Oh God, I forgot to return my agent's call!

The CAT scan machine covered me, protected me, it seemed, from the very service it was performing. I was a temporary guest within its confines. It would soon release me with a genial sigh, as if to say, "I can't imagine who sent you here in the first place. You are just as healthy as can be." I would go home, needing only a slight repair. Just a little stitch. No cancer at all.

I actually drifted into a pleasant sleep while, in the corner, the technician, a petite Puerto Rican with a thick braid down her back, was having a long phone conversation with (I presumed) her beau.

About thirty minutes later the machine turned itself off, and I winked awake. Well, that hadn't been bad at all. A little respite, a restoring nap, a meditation.

The phone call was ending. "'Bye, I'll see you later. Bring the chips, and I'll get the salsa. I love you too."

Once again the world proceeds no matter what. She was making a date, and I had just had an examination for cancer. Well, who ever promised anything else? I suddenly realized I was hungry. A Mexican lunch would be perfect right now. X-ray machines, guacamole, refried beans, questions, anxiety, frozen margaritas, tacos, blood tests, boyfriends on the phone, love, chicken fajitas.

It was all one. It was beginning to make sense, like a piece of needlepoint, one stitch dependent upon the next, an overlapping of wool, each skein its own color, but all creating a piece: a bouquet of flowers, a cottage in a leafy dell, butterflies, a tiny figure under the trees. And mistakes, knots, ugly places, and wrong colors too. Months later my son would say, "Hey, Ma, it's just life."

"Miss Barrie, that's it." She leaned over and smiled. Her teeth were perfect, white, and dazzling. "You're finished." (Little did she know.) "How did you do? It wasn't awful, was it?"

She gently helped me sit up. Holding my back and knees, she started to swing me around and help me off the platform as if I were 102. I snatched her hand away and waved her off. I was not yet sold down the cancer river. I was experiencing no pain. I felt just fine. I did not want to be a sick person.

"I can do it, thank you."

She looked hurt but quickly drew back. "Whatever you say."

I was truly a monster.

Barbara Barrie

April 27, 1994
Columbia Presbyterian Hospital

Sonogram time. Cast of characters: one Specialist, Dr. Something-or-other, age about twelve, who looked just like Tom Sawyer; one Middle-aged Female Assistant, motherly, knowledgeable, capable; and me, The Patient.

Once more I was lying on my side, only this time, instead of a finger or two, it was a mechanical probe with a camera on the end that projected the whole rectal area onto a small screen that I was definitely not allowed to watch. It was fantastically uncomfortable, and each time the probe rounded a corner or bumped into a wall, I said, "Ow!"

You'd be surprised how much better I felt saying "Ow!" It takes the place of "dammit," "Oh, God," "Jesus!," or "Fuck you." So I could yell it a lot, and no one could be too offended.

Doctor: "Let's move it here. Miss Barrie, would you shift a little forward, please?" I rolled slightly off my hip to the left.

Assistant: "Ah-h-h-h."

Doctor: "Mm-m-m-m. Could you draw your left knee a little higher, please?" I did as I was told, the blue gown threatening to fall off my thighs.

Assistant: "See that?"

Doctor: "Oh, yes."

"Hello," I thought. "Hello. Here I am."

Assistant: "Should I go a little bit up there with the probe?"

Doctor: "Yes, please try."

Me: "OW-W-W-W-W!"

Doctor and *Assistant,* together: "Sorry."

Assistant (whispering): "Could it be a second stage . . . the break there in the wall?"

Doctor (whispering): "Yep."

"Hello. I can hear you," said my inner voice. The outer one was silent.

Doctor: "Now, Miss Barrie, I'm afraid this will be a bit painful, but it will only be for a second." Pause.

70

Me: "OW-W-W-W-W-W!"

Doctor and *Assistant:* "Sorry, sorry, sorry!"

Assistant (whispering): "See that? Third stage, do you think?"

Doctor: "Mm-m-m. Yes, look at the tissue."

Assistant: "Ah-h-h-h."

Doctor: "Now lean slightly to your right, Miss Barrie. Thank you."

Me: "OW-W-W-W . . . EEE!"

Doctor and *Assistant:* "Sorry."

Doctor: "Now slightly forward one more time. M-m-m-m. See *that?*"

Assistant: "Oh, yes."

Doctor (whispering): "Third stage, for sure."

Assistant: "Bear with us one more minute—we're almost finished."

Doctor (*REALLY* whispering): "It's through the wall."

Assistant (also *REALLY* whispering): "Third, right?"

Doctor (muttering, almost inaudible): "Yes."

Now I had done enough research to know that tumors were labeled first, second, or third stage. "First" means there's a good possibility of complete cure. "Second" is still hopeful. But "third" means big trouble, probable metastasis already and major, major surgery.

When I was finally allowed to sit up, I asked, "It's a third-stage tumor, right?"

They both look surprised. "Well . . . uh . . ." They glanced at each other. "Well, uh . . . maybe . . . ah, yes, could be the case."

"In this instance, what does that mean?"

The Tom Sawyer doctor leaned over and said reluctantly, "It means, we think, that the tumor has penetrated through the anal wall."

"You're saying that I will have to have a colostomy, right?"

The Motherly Assistant said, "Perhaps, but Dr. Kelly will tell you more."

No "perhaps." It was a definite. They left the room so I could dress. I was getting calmer and calmer. What else could I do? I couldn't go backward and have the bleeding checked earlier. Crying wouldn't help. Besides, I seemed unable to do that.

This operation would be a radical procedure, and my life would be forever changed. I would have multiple scars and a red bowel opening covered by some sort of bag. Well, it's better than dying. And there's a lot I wanted to do before they put me into an urn somewhere.

APRIL 27, 1994

Dr. Kelly folded his hands beneath his chin. "I was hoping we could hitch things up so that we can leave you a rectum. But the tumor is so low that there will be no bowel to attach it to. It has to come out, and that means . . ."

"A colostomy."

"Yes. But it's not the end of the world. You'll adjust to it. You won't have an odor. You'll learn to easily take care of it and do everything you've always done."

We were in the examining room again. He had wanted one more look, and wrapped in a paper gown, I was now sitting on the edge of the table.

"Except, Dr. Kelly, that I won't have an excuse to lock myself in the bathroom and read."

He laughed. "That's about it. But you can read in the living room, and you'll have a lot more time at your disposal."

"'Disposal.' That's the perfect word, Dr. Kelly."

We both stopped speaking. The room was quiet.

"Will you do it?" I asked.

He looked startled. "Do you want me to?"

"Yes. I just feel that you've done things so thoroughly up to now. None of these tests was ordered by the other doctor. I feel safe here."

I knew I should have asked how many procedures he had done before and how many of the patients had survived. I knew that I should go away, talk to Jay, think about it, and call later. But a minute ago I had made the decision. I felt I had done the right thing.

"If you're sure, I will," he said. "Do you want some time to think?"

"No. This is what I want to do."

"Okay. Call Angela, my secretary, and she'll schedule the procedure."

We shook hands. It was done.

CHAPTER 11

Should We Tell the Children?

Walking home along Columbus Avenue from our regular Tuesday night at the New York Philharmonic on a sensuous spring night, the trees knobby with buds, people already sitting in outdoor cafes:

"You know, Jay, I've never heard the 'Concerto for Orchestra' in a hall, only in recordings."

"Masur is clearly crazy about Bartok," he said.

"But from where we sit, so high up, it's like choreography, isn't it?" I asked. "One section hands over the melody to another section, the violin bows ending low, the trombones going up to take the next note . . ."

"Gorgeous," Jay said. "The orchestra danced. I could go right back and hear the whole thing again."

"And see the whole thing again," I said.

"Yep, exactly. Want some ice cream?"

"The no-fat, no-taste kind on Seventy-second Street?"

"What else?" He put his arm around my waist and kissed my forehead. We stopped to look in the window of a jewelry store. I leaned my head against his jacket. We seemed to have pushed aside the impending operation on May 2. It was just there, an irrevocable fact, like standing on the platform, waiting for the train to arrive.

We purchased small cups of the ersatz ice cream, coffee for me and Snickers for Jay. They both tasted exactly the same, but the coolness, or the "coolth," as Jay calls it, somehow cleared my head. When in doubt or facing the unknown, always eat ice cream.

At home Jay poured us some wine, and we sat on the window seat overlooking the west side of Manhattan. There was, for once, no pollution. The stars were cheerful and territorial in their spheres, the promise of a soft, bright day tomorrow. In the distance the planes floated in a holding pattern for Newark Airport. A helicopter flew so close that we could read the printing on the side: FUJI FILM.

"Why is that thing flying so late at night?" I asked.

"Can you read it, honey?"

"Yes," I said.

"That's why it's flying so late at night."

"Jay, I've been thinking," I said, pulling a soft afghan over us. "I've decided I won't tell Jane and Aaron any of this."

"Why not?"

"Because they know I've never believed in illness . . ."

"You believe in this one."

"Yeah, but how about the time Aaron phoned a friend in nursery school? Remember? He said, 'I have to come to thchool tomorrow.' [He had a classic lisp.] 'I have a cold, but my mommy doethent believe in colds, so she sayth I have to go to thchool.'"

Jay laughed. "He was funny. And you were awful about any of us being sick."

"Ironic, isn't it?" I said. "I couldn't tolerate illness, I've never been sick a day in my life, and what do I get? The Big C."

"Ho ho. Very ironic. But I told you, if you don't include them, they'll be extremely hurt, even angry, I should think."

"I could tell them but urge them not to come home."

"Barbara, you can't. That's got to be up to them." He stood up and began to fold the afghan.

"I've got to think about it for a day or two, Jay."

"Stop treating them like babies. We really should phone them tomorrow."

"I know, but . . ."

We finished our wine and put the glasses into the dishwasher. We walked slowly to our bedroom. Face washing, moisturizer, teeth brushing, Water Pik, floss, the gum thing with the rubber end, the eleven o'clock news . . . all the sixty-year-old tasks. Really, truly boring.

Then we climbed into our high four-poster, read our books, chatted occasionally, and turned out the lights. We lay on our backs, our hands touching.

"Jay, since I only have four days till D day, do you feel even . . . slightly in the mood?"

Long pause. "Honey, I'm sorry, but I don't think so."

"You're so upset . . ."

"I am." His throat caught, and he turned away. It was the first time I had seen him fall apart, but I didn't have the courage to ask him to talk. If he despaired, perhaps I didn't want to know about it. He seemed to be in a new, private place.

I knew his eyes would be full. Since the children had been born, he had cried easily at small things: GE commercials; good report cards; Aaron singing in the choir at our temple, Rodeph Sholom; Jane, at five, dancing in her tutu and tiara. And this cancer, I suddenly admitted, was absolutely, utterly, irrevocably, the most ferocious crisis we had ever faced.

Okay, tomorrow we would call Jane and Aaron.

I kissed his shoulder. I wasn't hurt at his not wanting to make love, only disappointed. I must leave him alone to deal with his fears and sorrow. Oddly enough, I felt that I'd be all right, that having a colostomy was better than being in pain, a slave to the bathroom. That there might be a cure for my long-bothersome condition was hopeful to me, even there in the dark on that tender spring night.

But when would we make love again? What if I died during the operation and this would have been the last time?

The strange, maddening psyche: My body, with its aggressive, angry tumor inside, was alive and ultrasensitive. I longed to be touched. Everything felt erotic: the cotton sheets, the soft air, the skin of my breasts and thighs, even the soles of my feet. I wanted to have my fingers massaged, my ears kissed. I wanted to pull Jay up to his knees and throw my arms around him, really hard, and push my body against his.

Maybe it was my affirmation of life, or maybe I *needed* an affirmation of life. But Jay was afraid, almost grieving.

In the dark, with the city lights diminishing below our window, I was in the bare-bones motel on the first morning of our honeymoon, over thirty years ago. I am a low blood pressure zombie in the morning, so Jay got up first and went to find take-out cups of hot coffee—an act of such generosity that I was amazed at the modesty with which he accomplished it.

"Here's your fix," he said as he poured in the milk. He climbed back into bed, and we drank our coffees together. We were easy and comfortable, as if this had always been our morning routine. (Actually it has become our ritual for thirty-three years.) Then we discussed every detail of yesterday's wedding in the elegant, manicured garden overlooking Lake Michigan.

"You were totally green," I said. "All day."

"I know. I looked into the mirror once, and this Green Giant face appeared. A Green Giant with a receding hairline."

"Oh, stop that. It's not receding."

"You're blinded by love, Barbara." He kissed my cheek.

"And I cried so hard during the ceremony," I said. "What got into me?" I leaned my head on his shoulder.

"Maybe you were regretting it?" he asked.

"Of course," I said. "I only waited twelve years for yesterday, but I do think I was scared. A weighty moment. I mean, that was a really weighty moment."

"It better have been," he said.

We watched the morning news, and then we made love. We went swimming in the motel pool filled with kids shouting and exuberant as they whooshed down the bright blue slide. We had pancakes and fruit at the outdoor Formica counter, went back to our room, and made love again.

So tonight I gently rubbed his back until he fell asleep. And then, late, late, I finally closed my eyes and drifted into dreams of little blond children afloat on red lava streams bursting from a mammoth volcano.

CHAPTER 12

Phone Call to Kids

The next day we called Aaron's apartment in Santa Monica, where I knew he and Jane would be doing their homework for the new sitcom. They were also preparing a "spec" script for "Roseanne."

Jane was twenty-eight years old at the time. She's streaky-blond, smart, slim, and totally organized. Aaron, twenty-five, is loose-limbed, athletic, intuitive about people and emotions, almost as if his cells are made of extrasensory material. I knew he would probably still be in his torn pajamas, walking around, acting various characters, improvising and asking questions.

Jane improvised with him while manning the word processor, economical in her movements, getting it all down on the screen no matter how theatrical the moments became. Together they hammered out every plot, every character, every word, every comma, every dash. Aaron would keep talking as he made fresh coffee in the kitchen. He'd bring Jane a cup, sometimes a piece of toast, and they'd work on through the California morning.

"Listen, Jane, wouldn't this guy say, 'Let's forget the restaurant'? I mean he's got other things on his mind."

"You mean the fact that his girl is pregnant? He's come to terms with that . . . he's hungry. He wants to eat."

"Yeah, but he's not a dork. She's in the room, for God's sake, he's not going to hurt her feelings."

"He's not hurting her feelings, Aaron. She's hungry too."

They'd laugh, then start the dialogue over, each taking a part. They'd screen the phone calls and answer the ones they deemed necessary. Aaron would stretch and do some push-ups. Jane would flop on the couch, her long arms and legs splaying out like a rag doll's. In a few minutes they'd resume.

When the computer was turned off and the day's work printed out, they'd continue their ingrained, constant sibling rivalry, which began the moment we brought Aaron home from the hospital, and Jane, aged two years and four months, cried, "Take him back!" (I know this sounds too pat to be true, but that's precisely what she said. And she maintained it, stomping about in bewildering despair until three o'clock in the morning, when she finally fell asleep in my arms.)

In the summer of 1993, I had been shooting a television episode in Lòs Angeles and came one day to pick them up for lunch. As I approached the front door of his little bungalow, I heard Jane say, "Aaron, are you ever going to clean this apartment?"

"Chill out, Jane. Concentrate on something important."

"This is important. Can't you at least get rid of that pile of laundry in the middle of the bathroom floor?"

"It's my apartment. You don't live here."

"But I have to work here. It's disgusting!"

And on and on . . .

But now we placed the call. Jay was on the other phone in the bedroom, and I, oddly calm, waited for them to answer.

Aaron answered. "Hi, Mom, what's up?"

"Is Jane there?" I asked. "We have some news."

"We? Should I make this a conference call?"

"Yes, please," said Jay. "How are you, honey?"

"Fine, Dad. Hold on now till I hit a button."

"Hi, Mom." It was Jane.

"Hi, Jane," we said.

"What's the news?" Aaron asked, softly. He sensed something was about to happen.

"Well, there's good news and bad news," Jay said.

"Give us the bad news first." Jane, ever practical and wisely self-protective.

"It seems that I have a little bit of cancer."

"What?" they both said together. "What are you talking about?"

"I was diagnosed a couple of weeks ago, and I've been getting opinions."

"What kind of cancer?" Aaron asked, trying to be sensible and unpanicked. I could feel Jane becoming very quiet, as she does when she's trying not to cry.

"It's . . ." I paused, "cancer of the rectum." Even as I said it, I remained unperturbed. This had happened, hadn't it? Jay and I had concluded that we had no choice but to relay the news. I was not going to die, I really believed that, so I must talk to my children and try to communicate my feelings.

"Oh, my God! What do they do about it?" Aaron asked.

"First they take the tumor out," Jay said.

"And then," I said, as quietly as I could, "they take out the rectum."

Aaron made a choking sound. "Mom, how can that be?"

"It's done all the time, Aaron. I'll feel so much better when it's all over. It's a fairly common cancer, and the prognosis is good, it really is. You must believe me."

"Oh, Mom, are you terribly upset?" Aaron's voice was full of concern.

"Mommy, how's your spirit?" whispered Jane. She was fighting fear, I could hear it.

"I don't think it's quite hit me yet. But, you know, it's a kind of relief."

"Relief?" they both repeated.

"Yes. It's as if the other shoe has finally dropped—I've always had so much trouble in that area, as you know."

"You mean all those hours in the bathroom?" asked Aaron.

"Yeah, that and a lot of other things," I said, not wanting to go into details that might further upset them.

"Well, I don't get it," said Aaron. "How will you sh—, I mean . . . ?"

"How will I defecate?" A little vocabulary lesson in the midst of a crisis.

"Oh, yes . . . good word, Mom," said Aaron. He was trying to lighten up too. "How will you . . . defecate?"

"They redirect the bowel so that it comes out on the abdomen," I said, as casually as I could. It didn't work.

"On the belly?" he yelled. Jane gasped, then grew more silent than before.

"Yes," said Jay. "Mom's cousin Caroline had the operation a few years ago, as elective surgery, and says for the first time in her life she's free of pain."

"Where on the abdomen, Mom?" asked Aaron.

I was at last glad to be imparting this information. To me it represented future health, disappearance of pain, and I hoped that I could make them understand that there might be a cure and that I was willing to take the chance. "Probably on the lower left-hand side, Aaron," I said, "around the level of the belly button. But every doctor does it a little differently."

"What's the doctor's name?"

"John Kelly," said Jay. "Jane, are you there?"

"Yes, she's here," said Aaron, too quickly. "She's fine."

No answer from Jane. "Janie dear, now don't be upset," I said. "This is actually a blessing in disguise."

"You're kidding, Mom, right?" Aaron's voice was firm and steady.

"Mom's been sick and didn't know it," Jay said. I felt a rush of guilt. I had known it for a long time. Why couldn't I tell them that I had been in denial? For some reason I was too ashamed, and I said nothing.

"Kids, I'm going to be strong again, and the prognosis is excellent," I said. "They say that if you're going to have cancer, this is a good one to get."

"Oh, sure," Aaron said. "And the operation is called a what?"

"A colostomy," I replied.

"I've read about this. You'll have to wear a bag!" Jane was back. "Is that the good news?"

"Well, in a way," I said. "I won't always have to scout out the public bathrooms, and for once I might not always be cramping and uncomfortable."

"Were you always that way?" asked Jane. "Why didn't you ever tell us?"

"Well, I guess I wanted to keep it secret. I wasn't too thrilled to feel so damaged, you know."

"What kind of bag, Mom?" asked Aaron.

"I haven't even seen it yet . . . a plastic bag, to . . . um . . . catch the [this was suddenly very difficult] . . . like a Baggie, I should think."

Now no one, from either coast, uttered a word.

Finally from Jane: "How does it stay on your body?"

"I have to confess that I don't even know. I guess I've been avoiding that part of it."

"Mom?" Aaron sounded very solemn.

"Yes, honey?"

"Will it be a Vuitton bag?"

My son, the comedy writer. A great line of dialogue through the darkening clouds. We all laughed for a long time.

"Of course," I said. "Only the best for me."

"When's the operation?" Jane asked.

"Monday, May 2."

"You're kidding. That's three days away!" cried Jane. "We're coming home."

"No, I don't want you to," I said, adamantly. I really meant this. I saw no reason for them to sit around the hospital and wait, then watch me come out of the anesthesia like a blob, messy and incoherent. "It is absolutely not necessary."

"Don't listen to your mother," Jay said. "It should be your decision. Whatever you do will be okay with us."

"We're coming," they shouted. "Tomorrow."

*   *   *

Now that is what I thought I heard them say, and it's what I first wrote when reconstructing the story. In actuality what they said was, "Okay, if you really feel that way." I had convinced them that it was a minor event and that I would be healthier than before.

I didn't discover until a year later that my sister-in-law, Margery Harnick, had called them the next day and said, "Kids, your mom is really sick. You've got to come home." Jane phoned American Airlines, which gave her an "emergency fare" immediately. A day later, to my complete amazement, they walked into the apartment.

Since then I have pondered my decisions over and over. Jay had been sure that first day we had phoned Santa Monica, that I had done the right thing. What I had not done was tell them all the ramifications.

Aaron recently said, "If someone has older parents, which I do, the least they can let you do is come along for the ride. And if they don't, then it's not really a family, is it?"

"Aaron, I had no fear of dying then," I said. We were sitting in a Los Angeles restaurant. "I would have told you if I had known how serious the operation was going to be. I just didn't understand it."

He leaned angrily across the table. "What's important, Ma? An opening night, a dinner party, or family unity? You said you had 'a little bit of cancer.' That should be the title of your book, *A Little Bit of Cancer*."

It's true that I hadn't wanted to frighten them. After all, the thought of losing a parent is one of life's most unthinkable traumas.

Ah. A lightbulb glimmered above my head one day as I was buying shoes on Columbus Avenue. My father died of a heart attack when I was fifteen years old. Could that have been the reason I had held back? Every day of my life I've thought of my sad, powerful father, a Latin scholar in love with Shakespeare, Coleridge, Yeats, Beethoven, and Brahms. I had wanted to spare my children even the idea that I might not make it, although I was absolutely sure that I would.

And in addition, had I not brought about this cancer? Had I not been bleeding badly for a year? Had I not refused to believe it was anything besides hemorrhoids? Why should my destructive behavior be foisted upon Jane and Aaron?

"Oh, Barbara, come on," Jay said one night as we were walking home from the movies. "You didn't do this to yourself. This cancer happens. Why are you dwelling on it?" His voice was harsh, annoyed.

"Because I knew, Jay, I knew," I answered, as we stopped at Fairway to buy some fruit for breakfast. "One day on Seventy-second Street I said to myself, 'Something is really wrong. I'm so exhausted that I'm having trouble putting one foot in front of the other. I'm horribly depressed. I've got to call the doctor.' But I put it off until I practically fell down in Charleston, until the cancer had leeched into a lymph node. How could I have been so crazy? You knew, though, that I was bleeding. I told you."

"Yes," he answered, "but not really how bad it was. I wish you had."

"Me too."

"During that time did you tell Jeffrey?"

No, I had kept it from my therapist-friend, Dr. Jeffrey Kramer, too. He'd put me on Prozac because I was beginning to go out of control in public, crying in the park, in stores, on the street. Evidently I was doing well physically, but mentally I was not strong enough to handle the stress of my life at that point.

After the diagnosis, Jeffrey had said, "It's fascinating, Barbara. There are studies now that pretty well conclude that depression can be one of the signs of cancer. You probably were sick for much longer than either of us could have imagined."

But I had refused to speak of my symptoms and suspicions. I had read enough about colon cancer that the thought of a perpetual bag on my hip, I now realize, was so repellent that I had gone into total denial.

But perhaps there was more. I was writing, I was acting, Jay and I had a vital social life, we constantly went to the theater and to musical events, the kids were creatively employed. I hadn't wanted anything to change.

And if there were a change, would I have had to face things that were not so wonderful? Those elements in any marriage, in any life, that one learns to accommodate? The hassles and obstacles that erupt all the time? I was afraid to examine them, but I was forced, by the depression, to do something. There were phantoms and ghosts, the Furies of Orestes, pursuing me through the parks, up and down the avenues, in my home.

As I was recuperating, Jeffrey and I had fairly regular sessions. One day, about six months after the operation, I had walked in seemingly calm and, for a change, fairly reasonable, but as the hour progressed, I found myself twisted with weeping. There were tissues all over the floor, the effects of the Prozac seeming to have vanished.

We had once more spent a lot of time discussing my denial of the cancer. "Barbara, let's talk about this again," Jeff said. "Why do you think you wouldn't admit to this illness?"

"I don't know," I sobbed. "I don't know."

"You may know more than you think. Try."

"I don't know. How can I know? I was afraid; I was ashamed. What could I have been thinking?"

"Go on."

"Well, if I didn't tell anyone . . ."

"Yes?" he asked.

"If I didn't admit it or tell anyone, maybe . . ."

"Maybe what?"

"Maybe I would . . ."

"What?"

". . . uh, uh . . . oh God . . . I would . . . *die*," I howled and buried my face in my hands."

"And then what, Barbara?" His voice was steady and supportive.

"Oh, Jeffrey, I would see my father. I'd be with my father."

"Yes?" He remained leaning back in his chair, totally still, as if any movement might alter this journey I was taking.

"And then I could tell him how sorry I was that I hadn't been a better daughter, that I hated his dying so soon."

The room whirled into a kaleidoscope of colors and images. The bookcases and chairs, Jeffrey's computer, seemed to float like objects in a Chagall painting; and I was there too, tilted, flying in the air, my hair hanging upside down. I was bloated with grief, but I had blundered into something. I couldn't stop crying.

"And what else?" asked Jeff, very softly.

I was choking. Where were the words? "And I could live with him forever. In the sky." I could barely talk now. "'Lucy in the Sky with Diamonds.'"

I stared at Jeff. He handed me a tissue.

"Good girl," he said.

CHAPTER 13

First Night, Hospital

MAY 1, 1994
COLUMBIA PRESBYTERIAN HOSPITAL

The colon and rectum make up the final portion of the digestive tract. Here water is absorbed from food digested by the stomach and small intestine. Food is then passed into the rectum and eliminated through the anus. Ostomates are people who wear pouches to catch their body wastes when this process has been interrupted. A permanent colostomy is often done for cancers of the rectum. An ileostomy, often prescribed because of ulcerative colitis or Crohn's disease or familial polyposis (just what it sounds like), is an opening leading into the small intestine (small bowel), which is higher up in the digestive tract.

A urostomy (a urinary diversion with a stoma) is also called an ileal conduit. All these procedures are rerouted to an opening on the belly.

There are over seven hundred thousand ostomates in the United States and Canada, and there are hundreds of thousands more in the rest of the world. Of these, many are children born without a rectum or with bladder/urological abnormalities. If these children are able to receive proper medical attention, they can go on to lead normal, healthy lives. But that care, alas, is not always available, and many of them do not survive.

The American Cancer Society estimates that there will be 1,359,150 new cases of cancer diagnosed each year. Among those will be 133,500 new cases of colon cancer and 39,000 of rectal cancer. A total of 554,740 people, with all kinds of cancer, will die, more than 1,500 people a day.

Signs and symptoms: rectal bleeding, blood in the stool, a change in bowel habits. It is a disease that runs in families, although other risk factors are high-fat, low-fiber diets and lack of physical exercise.

Detection can be made through digital examination in the doctor's office, sigmoidoscopy (a hollow, lighted tube to inspect the rectum and lower colon), or a stool test done at home, with strips of paper, and returned to the doctor's office.

If any of these tests reveal possible problems, more extensive tests, such as colonoscopy (examination of the entire colon with a tube-attached probe, which projects onto a screen), and a barium enema (an X-ray procedure in which the intestines are viewed) may be needed. (I've had a lot of barium tests in hospitals. A machine photographs you as you assume all sorts of naked, barium-sloppy positions on the table while lots of people are watching and taking notes. An ugly experience.)

Treatment for colon cancer: surgery to remove the tumor and reattach the bowel, and radiation. The jury is still out on the subject of chemotherapy for advanced-case patients, but combinations of "chemotherapy and immunologic agents" may help (postoperative) patients whose cancer has spread into the lymph nodes.

The American Cancer Society also says that colostomy is "seldom needed for colon cancer and is infrequently required for rectal cancer."

Didn't I get lucky?

I was going to have a colostomy—tomorrow, May 2, 1994—and there was no other choice.

I had been given a very small, single room at the hospital. I loved it. I didn't have to have a roommate.

Jane, a neatnik to set world records, organized the few things I had brought: toothbrush, books, face cream (God forbid I should be without it), dental retainer box (I have worn a retainer for thirty-five years), and a cotton robe.

Aaron made phone calls, his legs propped on the windowsill, to his latest girlfriend and to his best friend from college, Mike Rego, with whom he was forming a theatrical production company. Once in a while he or Jane would come to the side of the bed and give me a quick touch or a kiss.

I knew I should be agitated, frightened, but, again, I was possessed with a sense of inexplicable calm. Perhaps after the operation I'd be able to plunge on with my life with far less discomfort and no more worries about cancer. The Serpent had finally landed in my body, something I had thought for years might happen.

Now it would be like giving up smoking: Once I had really licked it, I wouldn't have to think about it anymore.

I sat in my bed and watched the scene play out around me. Jay, trying to be controlled, read a script and joined in occasionally with one of his wry bon mots. The kids, attempting to lighten the atmosphere, made truly obscene jokes, and we all laughed and talked.

The attending nurse was a large, well-proportioned bleached blond named Doris, about sixty years old. She was also a character. We learned about her two husbands, her journey to the United States from her birthplace, Vienna, and her other patients with colon cancer who had survived and were living normal lives. We all nodded our heads. That sounded like very good karma indeed.

"Well, darling," said Doris, bustling in with a gigantic white bottle, "here's your Golytely. Know how to use it?"

"Yes, all too well."

"Horrible, isn't it?"

"You have no idea unless you've actually had to drink it," I said.

"Oh, listen, listen, I had colon cancer."

"What?" We all looked at her.

"Oh sure, sure," she said, pouring my first disgusting dose. "Had the operation done right here in this hospital."

"Did you have a colostomy?" Jay asked.

"No," she said cheerfully, "but it was very serious. A big tumor. Radiation, chemotherapy. All that stuff. Lots of Golytely, all the tests, the bleeding. And look at me! Fat and sassy. In love. Nice, eh?"

"Married?" I asked.

"Oh God, dear, no marriage. I did that twice before, I wouldn't do it again. A very sexy guy. My age, but very sexy. He keeps his apartment, I keep mine." She held out a paper cup. "Now, Miss Barrie, you've got to start drinking."

I forced down a few gulps. It was the familiar taste: like aluminum, thick and pasty.

"No, come on, all the way down." I grimaced and felt my throat contract as I drank some more. "Uh-huh, that's the way. So this guy gambles, you see. Well, my husband did, too, that's why I kicked him out. But this one I'm not married to. He can throw his money away, but not mine. It works out just fine."

She filled the cup again. "More, dear, drink some more. Yep, that's good. Well, I finally got smart. I got just the arrangement I want. Now keep drinking this. Might as well get it over with." She placed the bottle nearer to me on the bed table. "'Bye for now. I'll be back to check on you," she said as she swung out of the room.

"Mom, really swig it," said Aaron. "Stop sipping, it just prolongs the inevitable." Pretending it was vodka and orange juice, I took a long drink.

"Oh, I'm going to throw up."

"Barbara," said Aaron, "you've got to throw up out of the other end."

"I'm trying, I'm trying," I said, hoping I sounded like Jack Benny.

If this seems a trifle theatrical, I have to admit that we are, as a family, very theatrical. Nothing is downplayed when it can be up-played. No joke or pun is left unexplored by Jay, whose face takes on a specific look when he's about to be witty, and we all cry, "Here it comes!" Hands go dramatically to foreheads when we talk; I cry "at card tricks," as Jay says; the children can assume tragic Barrymore-like stances in a moment and be witheringly funny in the next. We get angrier than angry and more loving than loving. And we say just about anything to each other, most holds not barred.

My children have no hesitation or embarrassment about bodily functions. Having been brought up in a Victorian household, I am always amazed what a normal, ho-hum attitude Jane and Aaron and their friends have about such things. If, as a girl, I had ever said "penis" or "vagina," or even "bathroom" instead of "rest room," I'm sure my mother's eyes would have rolled back in her head, and she would have fainted. Or sent me out of the house.

Now my stomach began to make aggressive noises, and I fled to the bathroom. "Wow. This is awful." My voice bounced off the pink tiles.

"Keep going, Mom," yelled Jane. "Fight the good fight!" She was the cheerleader yelling for the team, but through the door I could hear the effort it took. A wonderful actress, she was playing a difficult role. A role for her mom.

"We're behind you, Ma," called Aaron. "Pardon the pun."

In Jay's laugh there was relief that they were both helping him to find a sense of gaiety, to make me feel that all of this would be all right, that I'd survive. He'd been dealing with me alone for some time. Now he had companions, people he loved.

"You're very fresh, Aaron," I shouted back. "I'm your mother, and I have cancer."

You'd think that would quiet them down, but they all began to act like street kids, saying ribald, rude things to me through the door. When I finally emerged, they stared at me, their eyes twinkling, but behind the smiles was concern. What was happening to Barbara?

I drank more of the nauseating brew as we talked. Then I'd rush into the bathroom, screech and swear—they'd make their outrageous jokes, and I'd stagger back into the room. Every twenty minutes or so the whole routine would be repeated. I admired their tenacity. No one went home, they kept urging me on to victory, and it was now after two o'clock in the morning.

"I want to go to sleep, you guys. Please get out of here. I can't drink any more of this stuff."

"You don't have to. That's enough." Doris had silently white-shoed herself into the room. "Everybody out! We'll see you tomorrow."

More jokes as they put on their sweaters. I was really unsteady now and longing for some solitude. I mean, I adored all three of them, but I wanted some "alone" time, and I knew they had to be emotionally and physically depleted. Jane plumped my pillows, Aaron rubbed my feet through the basket-weave blanket, and Jay leaned over, ran his hand through my hair, and kissed me softly.

As they entered the little foyer and I couldn't see them, Aaron called back, "Tomorrow—new life, Barbara."

"And new tushy, Mom," said Jane.

"Good night, darling," said Jay, peeking around the corner. "See you in the morning."

I could hear laughter as the three pairs of sneakers squeaked down the hall. They couldn't fool me. I knew that by this time Jay would have one arm around each of our children, holding them close.

CHAPTER 14

The ICU

There were lights swimming on the ceiling, faint voices all around. Farther away, people yelling at each other, then laughing. A lot of things humming, clicking, flashing, and thumping.

I was high above the ground on some tucked-in, cozy surface. I felt no pain. Indeed, I couldn't feel my body. Was it there? I had no desire to move my arms and legs. Was I paralyzed? Why was there so much constant noise?

Oh, yes. I had cancer, didn't I? And there was to be an operation. Was it over? Someone put something into my ear, like a little stick. What was that? Whispered words from close, bent-over faces. What language were they speaking? Another stick in my ear. Why did they keep doing that?

I must have slept for a while. When I woke, I could see whole figures now, women in white clothes and colored sweaters, a man who delivered something to the women. And there, on two chairs, were Jane and Aaron, sitting utterly still, like polite children in a William Merritt Chase painting. My beloved Chase. My beloved children.

"Is that you?" I croaked.

They walked to the foot of whatever it was I was lying on.

"Hey, Mom," said Aaron. "How'ya doing?"

"Mommy, we're here," said Jane. She was smiling. I must be okay.

"Did I have an operation?"

"You did," she said.

"Is it over?"

"It is, darling." Oh, there was Jay on my left side!

I turned, with a cranking, old-car sound from my neck (What was *that?*), and said, "How are you?"

"I'm fine," he said, "and so are you. Everyone's very pleased."

"Why can't I feel anything? Why am I floating in space?"

"You're still sedated," said one of the young women.

Whatever they had me on was better than my nightly vodka. I had to get the recipe.

Could this be a nurse? She appeared to be a high school cheerleader. What was she doing here?

"What are all these wires and things?"

"You're in intensive care," said the young-woman-nurse-cheerleader. "We're monitoring everything that happens to you."

"It feels like Star Wars," I said.

"Dr. Kelly said the operation went very well," said Jane.

"What is it that they keep putting into my ear?"

"A thermometer," said Aaron.

"In my ear?"

"That's the newest thing," said the nurse. "It's very accurate."

As if on cue, Jane and Aaron waved and backed out of the room. They must have sensed that it was time for Jay and me to be alone.

I could not move my limbs. My vision was blurry. Tubes and wires, attached to every muscle, joint, and orifice, vibrated as they measured and recorded my complete bodily functions into computers that winked and blinked at my right side. I was decorated with knobs, screws, lights, clips, and curlicued objects. I was unwashed, un-tooth-brushed, dripping with unknown skin moistures. Dried spittle was at the corners of my mouth. I was a total mess.

Jay bent down and kissed me. "Wanna fuck?" he asked.

CHAPTER 15

First Operation

Columbia Presbyterian Hospital, Second Day
in My New Room, after Two-Day Stay in ICU

In Toronto, in late April, I had played Meredith Baxter's mother in a Movie of the Week called *My Breast*. My character travels from Florida to New York because, during a telephone conversation with her daughter, she senses something is amiss.

An intrusive, controlling guest, I am finally told by Meredith that she has breast cancer, but that the operation was a success, and her doctor had said that he "got it all."

"That's what they said about your father," I reply, "and four months later we were putting him in the ground."

A really swell, sensitive mother.

Dr. Kelly, on his first visit to the ICU, had bent low over me, his face close to mine. "I got it all," he said proudly. Floating happily on the remains of the anesthesia, I could just barely nod my head, but his buoyant manner and satisfied smile meant that in his opinion all the cancer evident had been removed, that I was out of danger.

Now, four days later, he loped into my little hospital room, leaned against the wall, crossed his arms and said again, "I got it all."

The IV bottle dripping into my arm pulled against my skin as I tried to sit up. "Why is it, Dr. Kelly, that surgeons always say just that in movies and television, but the patient often dies later?" I hoped I had said this with humor, but he jerked as if a bullet had hit him.

"Well, in this case, I'm really pretty sure that I did get it all," he replied. "There was one lymph node involved, and I took that out too."

Thud. Bad news.

My heartbeat went into overdrive. "How do you know there weren't other nodes infected?"

"Because I looked at every single lymph node and at the liver and under and over everything, and I'm sure there was only one."

"You mean you actually can see all the lymph nodes with the naked eye?" I had visions of Dr. Kelly looking through my lymph nodes, one at a time, as if they were a chain of beads wound throughout my body.

"Absolutely. I feel and look at the whole system. All the rest of the nodes were clean, I'm sure of that."

But there *had* been one infected, nasty, invaded lymph node. A jumping-off point for a cancer progression that had already broken the bounds of the tumor and pushed through into my body. "Does that mean that I won't have to have radiation or chemotherapy?"

"Well, I imagine you'll have to have treatment, but that's up to the oncologist."

So there it was at last. I was going to have to do it all: the radiation and its aftereffects, the chemo and its accompanying nausea, hair loss, weakness, puffiness.

"In a few days we'll send in the oncologist, Dr. Anderson, to discuss all this."

"But you do believe I'll have to have radiation at least, right?"

He hesitated. "I think whatever the treatment, it will be preventive. But, look, I'm not the expert. The prognosis for this kind of operation is really good; why don't you wait and talk to Dr. Anderson?"

"I don't have a choice, do I?" I attempted a smile, but I could feel it crumbling on my face.

"Dr. Anderson will be here soon. And Terry Haus will come to see you too. She's a specialist in ostomy care, and she's unbelievable. Just great. She'll teach you everything you need to know about taking care of yourself."

He walked to the bed, patted my arm in a disengaged manner, and looking as if he were heading off to play college rugby, waved himself out of the room.

FIFTH DAY AFTER OPERATION

Dangling my feet, I had been sitting on the bed several times during each day. Now I was asked to walk. Easy. A cinch.

Jane and Aaron helped me to stand. I looked like a patient in a documentary about insane asylums: my white hair uncombed, knobby knees and weak feet wobbling in scruffy slippers, the striped hospital gown open in the back, exposing everything. Only at this point I didn't care.

Accompanied by the ever-present, sloshing urine bag and the IV pole tottering along behind, we started down the hall to the solarium, which seemed an impossible distance away. The children made disrespectful jokes about bodily functions and older people.

"Stop that. It hurts when I laugh. My stitches will come out. Stop it."

"Laughter heals, Mom. Go with it," Aaron said, his hand solid under my elbow. Jane supported the other side. They'd make another awful joke, and clutching each other, we'd just stop and howl, people glaring at us for making such a racket.

I couldn't believe my fragility. Each step took five minutes, or so it seemed. My feet, like Donald Duck flappers, felt unattached to my legs. Against the pulling of the belly and rectal stitches, I was bent over like the witch in a children's story.

When we returned, about a million hours later, I fell into a deep sleep.

SIXTH DAY

Next to my bed was a morphine drip on a stand. When the pain was too intense, I could press the little rubber ball and give myself a shot of the drug. The drip monitored itself, stopping when the dose was enough. It only helped for a while, although the children said, "Hey, Ma, you're really grooving on that stuff!"

No wonder. I was draining through tubes at what seemed every possible point. I had metal staples from under my belly button to the top of my pubis, the incision through which the gut had to be pulled to its new position on the left side of my navel. I was glad not to be able to see through the dressing. I just couldn't face the reality of a new, raw opening in my body.

The tumor had been removed from the rectum and so, alas, had the rectum. Very sad. I had lost part of my body, and it hurt like hell where they had entered, done the operation, and sewn the buttocks together. I felt as if someone had tied me up with burning leather thongs. It was painful to lie on my back, but it was impossible, because of the IV, to turn over.

I wasn't allowed to have any food or water for what would be twelve or thirteen days.

"No water at all?"

"No," said Dr. Kelly, "we have to be sure that the new bowel works. It has to heal before we can let anything pass through it. You can take a sip of water with the pills, but just a sip."

"How can people live without water?"

"You have the IV, which hydrates you. You're in no danger at all."

I began to dream of Jell-O. On blessed doses of Percodan or morphine, I would drift into troubled sleep and immediately see raspberry Jell-O in cubes, like the ones in the *Ladies Home Journal* ads. And ice cream: a frosty wineglass filled with coffee ice cream covered with chocolate sprinkles.

Each time I awoke, my lips were glued together from the dryness; my throat felt as if it were filled with mattress stuffing. But I couldn't drink. If I had to die from hunger or thirst, I would unhesitatingly choose hunger. Thirst is like being in Sartre's *No Exit:* There is no escape from the torture.

SEVENTH DAY

Theatreworks/USA, Jay's company, had five plays in development, three in rehearsal, and many companies just returning from tours all over the country. When he arrived at the hospital, we would speak for a while, and then, without warning, he would fall asleep, leaving me feeling utterly deserted.

"You mustn't try to come here every day, Jay. I'll be all right, and you're worn out." I was angry, but I wasn't able to tell him. I was fighting for my life, and he was asleep.

"Oh, you mean you don't like me snoring, with my mouth open, sprawled out on the chair? How *impatient* of you, darling." He smiled with pleasure at his clever pun.

"Well, I'm not too thrilled with that, to be sure, but I feel terrible that you have to schlep up here on the subway all the time."

"It's nothing, Barb, it's a little train ride. Big deal." And then he'd nod off for a short nap, his summer-damp shirt drying in the air-conditioning as he slept.

Many months later I said, "Jay, how did you feel those early days in the hospital when I was recovering from the surgery?"

"Why do you ask?"

"Because you were really out of it. At least that's how I felt. You came up to the hospital and passed out in the chair."

"I might have been napping, but I know you," he said. "I knew that you were having a very bad time, and when things accumulate, you need to vent, to have someone to listen to you. I wanted to be there for you."

"But did I complain or talk a lot about it?"

"Yeah, I think you did. Not constantly, but you'd tell me how the day had gone, what the doctors said, things like that."

"And how did you react then? Were you resentful at having to be there?"

"Honey, I don't think so. You know me, I never listen anyway, so how bad could it have been?"

I realize that his falling asleep may have been a way to escape the reality of the trauma we were suffering. Of course, now that I'm in remission, he still falls asleep all the time because he really does work so hard. The difference now is that I complain about it constantly.

EIGHTH DAY

A gaunt, disheveled, gray-faced man stood at my door. "Hello, Miss Barrie. I'm your oncologist, Dr. Anderson."

"Oh, how do you do? Come in, please."

He sat down. "We'll start your treatment after you've healed." No pleasant banter first? Ill at ease, nervous, this man seemed to be without any social graces at all.

"Will it be a long treatment?"

"Oh, probably. There was one node involved, you know."

"I know." That one damned node. Might as well be all of them, it sounded so bad. Once again my heartbeat took off into the stratosphere.

"It could always come back, Miss Barrie. Or just because one tumor goes away doesn't mean another one won't appear." He blew his nose into a rumpled, dirty handkerchief and looked out at the view.

My head became a smashed watermelon, bursting open, the insides spilling out. I yelped something and clutched my temple.

"Miss Barrie, are you all right?" No, I wasn't. Couldn't he see that? "Would you like to see a drawing of your tumor?"

"Well, I'd rather not . . ."

He took a small pad and pencil from his pocket and started to draw a brutal interpretation of the tumor. It looked like a torture instrument from an Hieronymus Bosch crowd scene. "Here is the tumor. It was removed from just about this point in your rectum. It had penetrated far into the anal wall, so . . ."

"Dr. Anderson, would you mind opening the window a little?" I knew I'd faint if I didn't get some air and if he didn't stop talking.

"Oh, are you warm? I think it's quite comfortable in here."

"Well, it's hard to hear the facts laid out so succinctly."

"I see." He walked around the bed and opened the window. The late sun had been throwing hot beams into the room. Now a slight murmur of air reduced the nausea in my throat and cooled the perspiration dripping down my forehead and behind my ears.

"Thank you."

"We'll change the subject, Miss Barrie. Let's talk about the radiation that precedes the chemotherapy. Actually you'll reenter the hospital and begin them both together for a five-day period."

"I have to check back in?"

"Oh, it's not bad. A little intense," he said, scratching the exposed area above his badly laundered white socks. "You may get some not-nice mouth sores . . ."

"Dr. Anderson . . ." I started to cry.

"Have I said something to upset you?"

"Yes. I'm just not ready to hear all this. Can we do it another time?"

He started to make peculiar sounds in his throat and glanced about as if seeking help. "Well, goodness, don't you want to know the truth?"

"No. Not now. No."

"Yes . . . well, yes." He jerked out of the chair, nearly knocking it over. "I'll call Dr. Kelly and see when we can arrange another meeting." He drew his white coat around him and looking even paler than when he arrived, backed himself out, like a suppliant at a Buddhist shrine, into the corridor.

I made sure that I would never see him again, ever.

NINTH DAY

I had banned all visitors except Jay and the children. I prefer to heal on my own. I needed the quiet of an empty room, my books, my moisturizer, Public Television, classical music from WQXR in New York, and Court TV.

I didn't want to play the role of cheery, optimistic hostess-in-the-bed. It would have been too tiring and hypocritical. I didn't want to be considered unemployable by my industry. And since we had told almost no one of the cancer, there were few phone calls, although, mysteriously, there were more than I had expected. If anyone asked where I was, my family just said, "Oh, she's off in California on a shoot."

We had, however, told our very close friends John and Bobbie Leigh and Bert and Letty Cottin Pogrebin. Bobbie, during one of our Chinese-noodle lunches, had said, "I won't tell anyone, and you shouldn't either, not until you feel able to do so."

"That gives me the courage to do as I planned. Thanks for the assurance," I said.

She leaned across the table, her dark eyes intense. "It's

your life, you have the right to handle it as you please. Your illness is just nobody's business." Bobbie's laserlike clarity about things has always given me a quicker focus than I can find myself. I was very grateful to her.

One day, right after the diagnosis, Letty and I set out on our usual walk in Central Park. I told her the news. Visibly shaken, she stopped suddenly behind the gardens of the Tavern on the Green.

"I'm honored that you told me," she said tremulously, "and of course, no one else will hear it."

"Now, Letty, don't be upset," I said, hugging her. "I really think I can beat this thing." And I had not one doubt that I could. From then on, she and Bobbie were my constant confidants, my stalwarts, my secret-sharers.

In the hospital, flowers had been arriving, and Jay confessed he had told a few people at his office and a few others at rehearsal. Well, that's all we needed to get the news out. I couldn't even be angry. I knew that sooner or later it would be common knowledge, but I was still attempting to soft-pedal the whole thing for as long as I could.

Jay came every other day now; absolving him from a daily visit seemed to lighten his mood. He was able to go to bed earlier and stopped looking so drained from the hot subway ride.

Jane and Aaron, still visiting from California, came to the hospital often. They'd unwrap hamburgers and french fries and milk shakes, their legs, in narrow, holey jeans, slung over the arms of the chairs.

The room would smell like a McDonald's, an ambience I never particularly loved, but now I was starving. I saw dancing in my head an Egg McMuffin on legs, accompanied by hot, black coffee, both objects singing like characters in an animated Disney film.

"How can you do that to me?" I said.

"Oh, Mom," said Jane, "I'm sorry. Don't look. I just really have to eat something."

"Mom," added Aaron, spreading catsup on his potatoes. "Aren't you concerned for your children's nutrition?"

"You are both wretches. I'm starving. I'm dying of thirst. I have cancer."

"No, you *had* cancer," Jane said, firmly. She wanted me to get it clear: I had been ill—I was now getting well. "Your attitude is everything, Mom. You have to be more positive."

"Okay, I promise," I said. "By the way, tell me what the doctor told you when the operation was finished. You've never said a word."

"Well, he came out and said, 'Harnick,' and we all stood up," said Aaron, tearing into his burger.

"Then he said that it had gone very well, that he thought he had gotten everything," added Jane, "and then we all got a little weepy."

"Daddy too?" I asked.

"Yeah," said Aaron. "It was the end of a long day, and we were pretty emotional."

Jane gave her french fries to Aaron and started to laugh.

"What's funny, Jane?" I asked.

"Oh, Dr. Kelly said that he had also taken out a lymph node, and Daddy said, 'Who told you that you could take out a lymph node?' And the doctor didn't get it at *all*, not at *all*."

We all started to giggle, and then a fierce burning ripped through my belly. I couldn't turn over because the stomach staples were pulling, and the IV still limited my movements. I pushed my morphine button and tried to breathe deeply.

Aaron stood up and came to the bedside. "That drug is great stuff, isn't it?"

"Are you telling me I'm using too much of it?"

"No, I'm just wondering how much pain you're in."

"Oh, honey, it could be worse," I said. His concerned gaze broke my heart. I was doing exactly what I hadn't wanted to do: make them worry about me.

These children, now in their twenties, handsome and bright, had once been part of my body. Often when I was pregnant, Jay and I used to lie in bed and watch an elbow or a knee move across my belly. The magazine or book I was reading would jump up, propelled underneath by these astounding, clear determinations of life—a swimming, growing child.

Jay would try to catch the whizzing bump and say many times, "I wonder who's in there?"

Jane and Aaron had been in there. They were looking at me now, eating their sandwiches, drinking Cokes, running up my hospital phone bill, filling the room with hope, fluffing up my pillows, and saying things like "Watch that morphine, Ma. You could turn out to be a junkie."

"Fat chance," I'd say. And we'd all shout exaggerated Ho-ho-hos, clutching our bellies like three fat Santa Clauses getting ready to slide down the chimney with toys.

TENTH DAY

Dr. J. Gregory Mears's straight gray hair was combed neatly, a part running across the right side. A pin-striped shirt and bow tie peeked from the V-neck of his starched coat. His brown loafers shone in the morning light. Arms serenely folded over a perfect, burnished belt; his eyes crinkled through the horn-rimmed glasses. He was tall, slim, shining with cleanliness. Central casting.

"Your prognosis is excellent, Miss Barrie. This operation, because the tumor was so low, has a ninety percent cure."

"That's surprising, isn't it?"

"Not at all." He sat down in the chair near the window. With the sailboats and the Hudson River as a backdrop, he now looked like an Andrew Wyeth portrait or even a Norman Rockwell. "Oddly enough," he continued, "if you're going to have cancer of the colon or rectum, the rectum is preferable."

"Dr. Mears, give me a break."

"I'm serious. The numbers are just better."

"But do I still have to have radiation and chemo?"

"Sure, but it's really preventive. We don't see anything else in there. We just want to make sure nothing's going to come back. The chemo you'll get is a very light dose. You won't lose your hair. Some people don't even feel an effect."

"Dr. Kelly said he got it all," I said. "You and I both know there is a chance of recurrence, don't we?"

Dr. Mears looked steadily into my eyes. "Yes, but if you make it to the two-year mark, we consider you free and clear."

"So the patient is always caught between the surgeon and the oncologist, right?"

A thoughtful pause, then a rueful smile. "That's about it."

So here I was. The surgeon tells me I'm cured, that his operative skills have saved my life. But the oncologist is admitting that it would be a long time before I could be considered "cured." I had visions of myself looking like Poor Pitiful Pearl, being pulled apart by the arms, a doctor on each side.

Finally, "I guess I can absorb that, after a while."

"I'm sure you can," said Dr. Mears. I loved the fact that he didn't appear to have to leave, that he seemed prepared to stay until we had established some kind of understanding. "Your attitude is fine," he said. "Keep asking questions. I'm always available. It's not going to be as bad as you think."

"I'm glad Dr. Kelly called you," I said. "I guess you heard I had a little trouble the first time around with Dr. What's-His-Name."

"Yes, but that happens sometimes. Personalities, you know." A very politic answer. The doctor fraternity.

We shook hands and he left. We had been talking for over an hour. I was reassured. Dr. Mears might be my hero on the white horse.

ELEVENTH DAY

By this time I was doing fast walking around the halls. My body and my legs finally felt as if they belonged together. I loved swinging my arms and taking big steps in a new robe my designer friend Nadya had given me. It was long, fastened with mother-of-pearl buttons and shot through with gold threads. Not appropriate at all for the chlorine-smelling corridors of the hospital, but I didn't care at all. I was moving!

Whizzing around a corner one day, I passed a familiar figure standing in the corridor. Who was that? I kept going on my fast-walk, arms pumping up and down, a slight sweat beading my hairline.

Then I turned around. There was Letty, her arms laden with a hefty pile of magazines. She held up her hand, like a citizen in *Frankenstein* warding off the Monster.

"I know you don't want visitors, I know this might make you angry, but I just can't stay away. I had to see you. Don't be annoyed, please. Don't send me away. I'm just not going to take your word for this—I think you need a good visit. And I can't *believe* you're speeding around like that."

I laughed. "I've been doing it for days, otherwise I was going to go crazy."

How lovely. Here was my friend determined to break through the barrier. And she had done it. I threw my arms around her and beaming at each other like schoolgirls, we walked back to my room.

For the next hour we communed. Really, that is the only word. Letty doesn't like to waste a minute on frivolity, although she is a very jolly soul. We talked of the cancer, of my reaction, her reaction, what the future might hold, our souls and spirits, what God might think about all this. We laughed and cried a little too. We spoke of our children, who had all grown up together and were still fast, intimate friends.

We gazed out at the boats making white streaks on the Hudson River. The phone rang once—another mutual friend. "What?" she said, "you have a visitor and you wouldn't let me come?" I explained, Letty and I both feeling very naughty, that this had been a complete surprise, but I'm not sure the hapless caller believed me.

Don't Die of Embarrassment

It was a felicitous afternoon, and it actually changed my disposition enormously. I hadn't realized until then how much I had missed outside companionship. And for the rest of the week, I was immersed in practically every magazine published, all gifts from Letty. I read about the latest in city politics, the football analyses, the newest books, and, thank God, what one must absolutely wear, on the body and on the face, for the coming winter season.

CHAPTER 16

Terry Haus

TWELFTH DAY

"Hello, hello, hello. I'm Terry Haus. Did anyone tell you I'd be around?"

"Yes, Dr. Kelly said you'd be here."

"Well, here I am."

She was round and bustling, with a face from the ads for travel in Ireland. Profoundly blue eyes, strawberry-blond hair, faint freckles, spectacular skin, and the sweetest smell of soap and vanilla-y cologne.

With a grunt she plopped down. "My knees. I have terrible knees," she laughed. Her small feet didn't even reach the floor. "You know, I just love you. I love your work. I still remember *One Potato, Two Potato,* and I adored 'Barney Miller.' I see you on cable all the time. You've always been so special, so real, like you're not really acting. How do you do that?"

"Well, I . . ."

"I never got to see *Company,* but I did see that thing you did with George Burns on TV . . . what was it called?"

"Oh God, I can't remember."

"It doesn't matter, it was superb. How are you feeling?"

"I think I'm okay."

"Better than that, I hear. Everyone says you're recovering so quickly." From somewhere within her white coat, a beep sounded. She fished awkwardly in her pocket, then looked at the calling number on the black beeper.

"Do you mind if I answer that?"

"Not at all."

With deep breaths she reached over and snared the phone, which was just a bit out of reach. "Hello, it's Terry. What's up? Oh, no, you can't give her that. I'll come down in a minute. Don't worry, we'll find another way." She hung up and kept the phone in her lap.

"Miss Barrie, did you see the Movie of the Week last Thursday, with . . . oh, what's her name?"

"I did," I said, "and I can't remember her name either because I'm an ancient person. And she used to live in my building, and her father was a friend of mine."

"She was fabulous, wasn't she? I get home from the hospital, you know, and my feet and knees are just killing me, so I turn on the tube and just zero out. I'm ashamed to say that I go to sleep with it on. My daughter's in the next room, but she can't hear it, so I don't feel guilty. Tyne Daly. It was Tyne Daly in that movie."

"You're right, it was!"

It was obvious that we were not going to talk about the colostomy or how to treat it or what my future might be. Terry Haus was relaxing me, making me feel that we had plenty of time to do everything. It was all so ordinary, she seemed to be saying, that we didn't have to even think about it right now.

"You have children too, yes?" she asked.

"Two. Twenty-five and twenty-eight."

"Boys?"

"Boy and a girl. Jane's older."

The beeper rang again. Terry looked at the calling number. "That's one of the nurses. I'll be seeing her in a moment." Back into the pocket went the beeper. "What do they do, your kids?" she asked.

"They write as a team for TV sitcoms."

"It's all in the family. That's fabulous. You must be proud."

"Oh, I am. I think they're having fun together, and they didn't always."

"What do you mean?" Terry asked.

I didn't want to burden her with new and arcane information, so I just said, "Sibling rivalry. All that, you know."

"Umm. And is your husband in the business too?"

"He's artistic director of a company that produces original plays and musicals for children."

"Is it nice to have everyone involved in the same things?"

"Well, not all the time. It's a very mean game, Terry. May I call you Terry?"

Her face looked up as she laughed. "Of course. What else would you call me?"

We talked of her four daughters. Two married; two single—one was a buyer for an offbeat catalog collection. "She has a wonderful eye for design, things that people will buy. She started as a secretary there and made a place for herself." Her niece was at Exeter, already looking for colleges.

"My husband and I separated when the girls were little. There I was, with no job and three kids to support. Things were tough. What would I do?"

"What did you do?"

"I went to nursing school."

"Just like that? Who took care of the girls?"

"I did, at night. Baby-sitters, friends, the whole thing. I knew I wanted to do something useful. So I did it." She laughed again, her clean, soapy smell perfuming the space between us.

"Wasn't that unbelievably hard? Weren't you tired all the time?"

"Sure. But I loved every bit of it." Again the beeper. Cheerily she noted the calling number. "Another doctor. Everybody's got a crisis today. I'll call him in a second."

"But choosing the ostomy field . . . ?"

"I knew there was a need for it. At school I could see that no one was paying any attention to it."

Don't Die of Embarrassment

"But it's a pretty ghastly, messy business, isn't it?"

"Oh, no, Barbara . . . may I call you Barbara?"

"Please do."

"Well, we all have to defecate. It's part of living. I deal with a few of its problems. It's the same as changing diapers. You changed your kids' diapers, right?"

"Of course. I'd heard stories about babies born with fearful birth defects," I said, "so I was thrilled that everything came out of the right place."

"That's how I felt too. So now I just help people to adjust to a new routine. It's just shit, after all."

"Oh . . ." There didn't seem to be a ready answer to that. "Are you still in pain?"

"Yes, but I don't know what it's from. It seems to get worse, not better."

"Let me take a look." I raised my gown. "Oh, it's the stitches. Everything's healing, and they need to come out. I'll take them out for you one day, you won't feel a thing. Turn over and let me see the back." Slowly I inched my way onto my left side.

"Perfect. Perfect. It looks beautiful." (How beautiful could a sewn-up tushy be?)

I rolled onto my back and rearranged the gown. "Are you going to teach me how to do all this stuff, I mean the bag and the cleaning?"

"Try 'pouch.' Everyone likes 'pouch' better. Don't you?"

"I don't know," I answered, feeling slightly chastised. "My children love calling me 'the bag lady.'"

She laughed. "Oh, kids. I'm telling you. Anyway, I'll be teaching you everything, but not today. It's too soon. But it's going to be easy as pie."

She puffed to her feet. "I've got to lose weight. Why do I keep resisting? Now listen, I'll pop in on you all the time. *Two of a Kind.* That was the name of the George Burns thing! *Two of a Kind.* And Robby Benson was in it, too, remember?"

"Now I do. We shot it in the steaming summer in Pasadena. What a memory you've got."

113

"I do actually. Well, I just adore the movies and television. Where was I? Oh, yes . . . I'll teach you to irrigate once a day . . ."

"Irrigate?"

"It's like giving yourself an enema . . ."

"God."

"No, listen, it's the only way. You control your body, not the other way around. You'll see. We'll take it in good time. No hurry."

Her beeper rang again. "I know who this is. One of the surgical residents wants me to come and help him with a new colostomy patient who's had too many botched operations. There's just nowhere for the stuff to go." She glanced into the mirror and straightened her hair. "I think we're going to have to hook him up to the wall. Now I really have to go. Isn't it great that I can do all this? Of course, I'm running, running all the time, but it's worth it."

She carefully put the chair back in its place. Her Irish smile beamed into the corners as she sailed out of the room, insistent beeps trilling from her flowing white coat, as if, like St. Francis, she was surrounded by chirping sparrows on a bright yellow, summer day.

One day the sound of firm steps in high heels clicked down the hall toward my room. Even from a distance, it was a stride full of exuberant life.

"Here's Marge Scannell," said Terry Haus, ushering in a very pretty, shortish woman of about forty-two. A pink carnation was pinned to the lapel of her black and white suit. "She's the one I told you about, who has a colostomy and promised to come and see you."

"Oh, yes," I murmured, none too delighted about being interrupted in my reading. "How do you do, Marge," I said and held out my hand. Was she going to extol the virtues of having a colostomy? I hoped not. I just wasn't in the mood, although Terry had taken out the staples on my belly the day before (miraculously, without a twinge) and I was feeling more mobile.

Marge stood easily at the foot of my bed. I could tell immediately that she was not going to pressure me or cheerfully lecture on what my life should be from now on. Obviously she had been in many hospital rooms before.

"Terry asked me to come and answer any questions you might have, but if this isn't a convenient time, I can always come back."

She was also clairvoyant. "No," I replied, lying. "It's very good of you to come, but I'm not sure what I want to ask."

"Would you like me to tell you a little of what happened to me?" she asked.

Well, actually I did, but I hated to admit it. She was so radiant and optimistic that she was irresistible. I didn't think, however, that she would be able to impart anything to me because she was so much younger: Her hair was still blond, her skin unlined, her blue eyes as sharp as stars.

Terry sat down in the chair and turned off her beeper. "Tell her, Marge, she'll be amazed," she said.

"I had cancer of the rectum, just like you—oh, do you mind that I know?"

"Not at all." I was sure that Terry had told her, and that was acceptable because, after all, it's Terry's mission in life, thank heavens, to make us all well.

"Well, I was just devastated, of course," she continued, "but I got through it. I even got married, and here I am."

"You're wearing a pouch?" I asked.

"Sure. Want to see it?"

I hesitated. It would be my first time to actually see a pouch on another human being. In fact, I had yet to see a pouch at all.

Marge casually pulled down a band of her skirt. There on her belly was a round plastic circle, about the size and substance of a ruffled jelly jar top. "This is it," she said, turning slightly toward the window so that I could get a side view.

"Here's the top and it's attached to a plastic circle right here, surrounding my stoma. Simple, isn't it?"

"Can you feel it?" I asked.

"No, but you know, I irrigate, so it's usually empty, and I just don't think about it much. I go to work every day, I live a very full life—I volunteer for the Colostomy Society . . ."

"Part of that is visiting people like you, Barbara," said Terry, beaming, "so that you know this can all be managed. Isn't Marge just great?"

Indeed she was. They both were, but I was still resistant. I wasn't sure I would be able to take all this. Marge gave me a view from the other side, as if walking down the runway at a fashion show. "You may prefer a different kind," she said. "I wear this because I only have to change the top; the little plastic circle stays in place for a few days at a time."

Terry said, "It saves the skin on your belly, Barbara. Later on, when you're ready, I'll show you all the other choices."

Marge put her skirt into place and smiled. "Now have you had enough, or should we go on?"

"Show her your little kit," said Terry, presiding like a mother hen over her two little chicks.

Unfastening her purse, she pulled out a flat, neat Baggie. "Here's what I carry every day," she said. "A fresh pouch and another Baggie, in case I have an accident, although that really rarely happens, and a prep pad to smooth over my skin and protect it. It's the first thing I put in my purse every morning."

Now those daily preparations made perfect sense—practical solutions to a real problem. "Marge, I have just one more question." Might as well go for a high score. "What about your sex life? Has it been affected?"

She lifted her arms like the Botticelli maiden and laughed deeply. "Oh, it's fabulous. Really, better than ever because I'm not sick anymore, and my husband is totally supportive. He doesn't even notice the pouch." She grabbed her handbag and came around the side of the bed. "In fact, he's double-parked downstairs, so I have to run. He's driving me to work, and we have to do an errand on the way. But here's my number, please call me any time of the day or night."

"Thank you," I said.

She put her hand on my pillow. "Listen, I know this all seems insurmountable right now. I went through it too. But I want you to know that you'll conquer it, your life is going to be wonderful, and you'll look back at this period as just a temporary thing."

I smiled. Although I wanted to be more effusive, I just couldn't completely respond. Knowing that I was going to have to deal with all these new elements had just walloped me. What I needed more than anything was to sleep, to have time to recover from this onslaught, to make it part of my unconscious so that it could later seep into my conscious mind and allow me to function.

That was the process by which I've always learned lines and changes in a role during rehearsals—I've napped in many a drafty theater lobby.

Joseph Papp, the director, once accused me of not being interested in exploring the incomparable, divine Viola during work on *Twelfth Night*.

"Joe," I had protested. "I love this part, but Aaron doesn't sleep through the night yet, and I'm a basket case in the morning. It's just going to take me a little longer to inhale Viola and make her my own."

His face rippled into tenderness. "Oh, yes, I remember," he said. "You wake up in the middle of the night and wonder why you're awake. You lie there and *then* you hear the baby turn over." Like a woolly bear, he took me into his arms. "I understand. Take your time, Barbara, sleep all you want. I know you'll get there."

Now as I shook Marge's hand and thanked her, my eyes were grainy with fatigue. Terry waved an ebullient good-bye, and both women left the room.

I turned on my side and passed out.

CHAPTER 17

Maggie

THIRTEENTH DAY

Each day I grew stronger, walked faster, and explored new hallways and entrances. I felt confident that I'd get back my muscle tone. Had I really begun to conquer this thing? Perhaps having a colostomy wasn't the impossibility I thought it would be.

Suddenly one afternoon something happened around the site of the surgery. A cramp, a gurgle, and the pouch began to slowly fill. Oh my God. It had finally happened. And it was utterly horrifying. This was how it worked? The discomfort, the sound, the watery gush? I was going to have to live with this for the rest of my life?

I turned back toward my room, tears rolling down my cheeks; and for some strange, prophetic reason Dr. Kelly was standing in the doorway.

"What's wrong, Barbara?"

"It's working," I cried. "The damn thing is working. What do I do?"

I banged my forehead against the wall. Maybe I could push away the pressure and the rush and the bag forever attached to my body. The colostomy would have been a bad dream. My body would function as before. The operation would be reversed. I didn't mind the cancer as much as I loathed the reality of what lay ahead. I sobbed.

"Barbara, this is the normal, healthy reaction. Everyone is shocked when the bowel starts to function." Dr. Kelly held me by the shoulders. "We can be happy that everything is working well. You can have your Jell-O now and juice. You've been begging for juice."

I smiled and kept weeping. Not an easy feat. "Oh, Jell-O. I'm saved." Then more tears. What a drag I must be. "But I don't know how to deal with the pouch or how to clean myself or when it's going to happen from moment to moment."

"That's what Terry Haus does. She'll come back now, right away. Meanwhile here's Maggie, our head nurse, and she'll show you the first steps, right, Maggie?"

"Oh, hon, don't worry," said Maggie. She was six feet tall with an exquisite face and black braids wound around her head like a crown. "Let's go into your bathroom. You're just having the natural response when the bowel starts up again. It's scary. Everyone feels this way." She extricated me from the folds of Dr. Kelly's coat.

"Sorry to be so difficult," I said. They both murmured and patted my shoulders. Dr. Kelly bid me a concerned good-bye; and like an elderly, passive invalid, I was led into my bathroom.

"Now just take everything off, and we'll change you [change me?] in a minute."

She began to gently pull off the cuff around the pouch. And then, for the first time, I saw the colostomy. It was protruding, red, and swollen around the edges, much larger than I had anticipated, like a miniature inner tube. The center closely resembled the spigot of a garden hose. Was it supposed to look like this? I turned my head away and held on to the toilet edges.

"I know it's a shock," said Maggie, as she swabbed my belly with a protective solution, "but it's new and raw. The edema will go away. This is not the way you're going to look."

I was gagging from the smell. She gave me a drink of water. "Put your head down, hon, keep it down."

I did as I was told, while whimpering like a malnourished kitten the entire time. Maggie kept handing me tissues and said, "I understand. Just stay that way for a few more minutes." She attached a new pouch, this one clipped with a plastic fastener at the bottom.

"What's this?" I asked.

"This is the drainable pouch. From now on we'll drain everything into the toilet and rinse the pouch through with water. Then we won't have to keep ripping at the skin around the opening."

This was worse than I could possibly have imagined. Why had they told me I could have a normal life? I would have to stay in my apartment forever, a recluse, an outcast, lonely and separated from society. I was desolate.

Maggie helped me into the room. She tucked me into bed and sat on the ledge under the window. "Hon, you'll laugh at this one day."

"How could I?"

"Oh, believe me, you will. You've been through a major operation, and this is the first time you've really given in to it. I see you racing around the halls, laughing with your kids. I know you won't even allow any other visitors. You're amazing, but sooner or later this was going to hit you, and today's the day."

"I'll say." But a "drainable" pouch? Was I always to be saddled with a half-clean bag? I soon found out that there are efficient, neat, throwaway bags, but at that moment I was afraid to ask anything.

Maggie had been a nurse for fifteen years, she told me. Her husband was a sculptor and painter. They had just come back from a vacation in the Caribbean, where he had worked, and they had walked the beaches and swum in the ocean.

"He's my second husband. The first marriage was a bummer. [Another nurse with a bad first husband.] But I had a great kid."

"Had?" I asked.

"Oh yeah, he was going off to Annapolis in August." She walked to the bed and briskly pulled the cuff of the sheet over the blanket. "He was shot dead in a gas station."

"Oh God, Maggie. When?"

"Just a year ago yesterday. They brought him into this hospital that night. That's why we went away. I couldn't face being here."

"How did it happen?"

She placed my slippers under the night table. "He was with some of his friends, and there was a robbery. They got caught in between, but he was the one who got the bullet. And he was my only one, my only baby."

I stared at her. "How have you survived. Just a year? How are you doing it?"

"Oh, you just do. Here, it's time for this pill." She placed two capsules in my hand and poured a glass of water from the metal pitcher. "I have my work, I have Judd, my husband. What am I gonna do? Give up? I came to the hospital the next week, I thought my heart was dead, broken, why was I living? Want some more water, Miss Barrie?"

"No, thank you."

She took the glass and rinsed it out. "But, you know, you get on with it. You don't have a choice."

I had stopped moaning. "I can't get over you," I said.

"Well, we all have our sadnesses. You have yours too."

"But it doesn't compare to yours, Maggie."

"Maybe not. But to you it does. It's your life, isn't it? But like I said, in a few months you won't even think about your operation. It'll be part of your daily routine, nothing more." She cranked up the foot of the bed. "Now just turn on the TV, hon, and rest for a while. You're going to be just peachy."

Peachier than she would be for a long, long time. I'm sure that you never get over the death of a child, you just learn to live with it. Maggie was doing that. Her strength and determination had been palpable in the room. George Bernard Shaw's *The Life Force.*

She had tried to impart some of it to me. I was humbled, grateful, in awe. Her only son had been murdered.

Who in the hell was I that I could have carried on like that?

CHAPTER 18

Home from the Hospital

When Jay brought me home from the hospital, our apartment seemed like a luxury hotel. Not that Columbia Presbyterian hadn't been terrific—I had looked out on the Hudson River from that small room. Sunsets, sailboats lilting toward West Point, and the moon pinpointing the lacy steel of the George Washington Bridge.

The renovation was technically complete, and everything was new: faucets, kitchen equipment, floors, doors, crown molding, bookshelves. Window seat cushions and bed curtains had not been delivered, but it was a real home now—a fresh, clean beginning after the large but cluttered apartment on West End Avenue. There was still a strange, gluey smell from the new cabinets in the living room, but dealing with a new plastic appliance attached to the left side of my belly and being somewhat in pain, I couldn't worry about it. However I did open the cabinet doors to let in fresh air (my children say I was born with a sponge in my hand) and collapsed onto the sofa. I was moving very slowly and awkwardly.

The consequences of this illness were gradually beginning to surface, a few thoughts at a time. What if the cancer popped up in another place, as it well might? How would the children react to such news? My husband was smart, handsome, and funny. He'd be fine, probably married within a short time. At least that's what I'd hope for him. I think.

I had not really considered dying: The thought hit me in

the hospital as I was struggling against the stitches that prevented me from sitting up. To be put under the ground in a box? What if I were still alive and no one knew?

I had drawn up my Living Will with David Dretzin, our lawyer. He and his wife, Joanna, two of our cherished friends, had shared a soul-food meal with us in the neighborhood on the night I had signed the papers.

"Please, David, be sure they don't attach me to some ghastly machine to keep me alive," I said. "I know we have the Living Will, but sometimes I hear they don't honor it."

"Barbara, I guarantee it, but don't forget you've appointed Margery and Sheldon as your proxies, so nothing like that is going to happen. You'll be back on the courts in two weeks." His kind face gave me great courage. I knew they would all protect me.

"I don't want anyone to know about this illness, okay?" I said.

In their typical, empathetic way, they had both nodded. "Not a soul will know," said Joanna, "but are you sure I can't take you to the hospital tomorrow? Can't I come to visit? We live so close, it's just a minute."

"I'll let you know if I get lonely," I promised, taking her hand, which immediately made her very watery. Everyone knows about Joanna: Her tears, particularly for friends and at weddings and funerals, are an inch below the surface and fly from there into the air and down her beautiful face.

After signing the papers, we clinked our beer bottles and ordered gooey, obscene desserts. We all hugged good-bye in front of our building, and everything seemed in place, hopeful. I was actually looking forward to getting on with the operation.

About five days after I returned from the hospital, I was watching "McNeil-Lehrer." For some inexplicable reason I suddenly realized, "Oh, my God, I may never see my grandchildren." That is, if either Jane or Aaron settled down and made me a happy, white-haired grandmother.

The five days of combined chemo and radiation lay ahead. Then radiation alone, a trip to the hospital every day for seven or eight weeks. Meanwhile here I was, looking like a famine victim: colorless face, bone-thin frame, stringy hair. Would I be able to go back to dance class? I was told the radiation would reduce my libido. Would I ever make love again? Would I ever want to make love again? My body felt like a cable-stitched sweater that had been hit by a speeding bus.

And what would happen to my tennis game? I had finally found my backhand again last summer on Fire Island. I was hitting better than ever, and now . . . could I even extend my front leg as the ball approached? I mean, my tushy was completely sewn up! Wouldn't it hurt? Would the stitches come out and the empty space that was now there be completely exposed—open, ripped, and agonizing?

And then, once more, would I die soon? Much sooner than I expected? I'd take seventy. Seventy would be a good number. Seventy-five was too much to hope for, and I didn't want to be like my mother at ninety-five: incontinent, angry, unable to read or watch television anymore, her short-term memory completely gone.

I didn't want the kids to have to watch me fade away in some cold hospital room, tubes in every orifice of my body. I didn't want to die the way my friend Louise had died—unknowing, so sick, belching forth a black liquid that her husband said he would never forget.

Yes, I'd take seventy. Maybe a heart attack in my sleep. No more chemotherapy after the year ahead of me. No more radiation, no more operations, no matter what they told me needed to come out. I would be brave like Jackie Kennedy, say no to any extreme measures, and hope and pray that at seventy I would go peacefully "into that good night."

After all, I had had a fabulous life; a wonderful career that had carried me around the world; a loving, talented husband; and two children who were like children from dreams. Jane—sharp and pretty, complicated, so interesting. And

Aaron—gentle, handsome, smart, and with an ESP that could snatch emotions and undercurrents from the air. True, we all had had problems with one another through the years—sometimes severe—but didn't all families?

That night, before going to bed, I had to change my pouch by myself for the first time. Gingerly pulling the tape that holds the pouch in place, I saw my body in the mirror. On the left side of my belly was a red, mouthlike aperture. Oh my God, it was the stoma, the opening of my own bowel pulled through the skin. My intestines blatantly exposed—glistening with moisture and actual feces. The secret functions of my colon and rectum no longer secret. The smell was a shock, the skin around the stoma oozing pus or mucus . . . I couldn't tell. And the sudden, burning, raw intensity was almost unendurable. I started to gag and held on to the sink, my eyes shut, trying to pretend it away.

At first I whimpered while trying to clean myself with a moistened piece of gauze. That only hurt worse, and I started to sob like a person deep in grief. Well, I was grieving—for my lost rectum; for the natural functions that were forever altered; for my smooth, flat stomach, now bumpy and scarred from above my navel to the center of my pubis. And because of the amazing, wild pain.

Jay called out, "Honey, honey, can I help?"

"No, I'm all right," I sobbed. (You can imagine how much he believed me.) I pressed a wet washcloth to the area. The pressure quieted things down. I gingerly dried the skin and applied the new pouch, which acted like a Baggie gone crazy. It puckered as I tried to smooth it around the stoma. It stuck on one side before I was ready for it to stick. From all the fumbling, too much air had entered it; suddenly there was a small, puffed balloon on my belly. I couldn't bear to rip it off and start over, so I emerged from the bathroom looking like a lopsided pregnant woman, spraying the "Med Spray" deodorant everywhere and throwing open all the windows.

Jay sat up in bed. "What the hell was going on in there?"

"It's a big adjustment. It's hard to come to terms with this."

"Honey, honey, it's only shit!" He looked stricken and pale and weary of the entire thing.

"I know. But there's the soreness—oh, I mustn't be a whiner."

"You're never a whiner, except when I'm late, and then you scream and make my life miserable."

"Very true."

"Come on, put your little headie down." (That's what we said to Jane when she was a toddler, and we wanted her to nap or sleep.) I smiled a pathetic smile and crawled under the sheets. Jay put his arms around me, and although I wanted to share this experience, I couldn't do it: It was too personal, too humiliating, too messy.

He was snoring almost immediately. Neither rain, nor snow, nor gloom of night could interfere with Jay's slumber. I turned off the lamp and lay on my elbow, staring into the dark. Soon the steady, insistent sound of the sleep machine filled the room. I pushed his shoulder and hissed, "Try to stop snoring, please."

"Gimme a kiss," he said, waking a little. I leaned over and kissed his cheek, then his mouth.

"'Night, honey," he sighed.

"Good night," I said and kissed his hair. As it was too uncomfortable on the left or right side, I fell asleep on my back, struggling with the desire to turn over and snuggle into a pillow.

And that was the end of my first day home.

This scene, I am embarrassed to say, was repeated almost every night for two weeks, until the pain eased and I could get used to disposing of my own feces. I had changed the diapers of the children, but they were of course my perfect angels. I was not an adored, perfect angel. And this procedure, accompanied by howling, crying, and swearing, certainly didn't make me one.

CHAPTER 19

Phone Call from Jim

A few days after coming home, when I was walking around the apartment again, the telephone jangled as I was preparing dinner. It was cousin Jimmy Boruszak from Chicago.

"Barbara, how are you?" He is a big, expansive man. His voice is the same.

"Fine, Jimmy, how are you?"

"Great, great. How's Jay?"

"Overworked. The Children's Theatre is time-consuming, but he loves it, so what can I do?"

"And the kids?"

There's no chair in our little kitchen, so I pulled over a little stool and gingerly sat down, a vodka-filled glass in my hand. "There's a lot of action on their pilot. The Fox network wants to hear it read, and they're working on a new pilot."

"What terrific news."

"Yes, we're thrilled for them."

"So, Bobs!" This was a lot of enthusiasm for a normal, cousin check-in."

"Yes, Jimmy?"

"You got the family disease!"

News travels fast.

"How did you find out?"

"Well, I don't know."

"I'll bet it was Sandra, wasn't it? She was here when I was

in the hospital, and Jay had to tell her because I didn't want to see anyone."

"Bobs, I really can't remember. In this family do you think you can keep any secrets?"

"I don't anymore." Some nagging twinge of dread was swiveling into my head. "But, you know, I didn't have irritable bowel syndrome or colitis or diverticulosis. What do you mean, 'family disease'?"

"Well, cancer. We have a history of intestinal problems, but cancer is the disease. You knew that."

My hand began to shake slightly, the ice tinkling against the side of the glass. "I knew your dad had cancer, but was it this kind?"

"Are you kidding? Of course. What did you think?"

My funny, volatile Uncle Burt. Oh my heart. "Well, no. When he died . . . how old was he, Jim?"

"Fifty-seven."

"Oh God, he was so young."

Jimmy's voice lowered. "Yes," he said. "Yes, he was."

"I didn't know. In those days no one talked openly about cancer. I mean, it was all whispers and secrets, wasn't it?" I asked.

"Not to us. Didn't anyone tell you when you came to the funeral in Chicago that Dad had cancer of the colon?"

"I don't remember. Was that in 1958?"

"Yes."

"Maybe someone did," I said, "but I must have forgotten. Or wanted to forget."

"My God, Barbara, I have an examination every year. I'm fanatic about it. I saw how Dad suffered. I'm not going to let that happen to me. Caroline [our second cousin] had surgery a few years ago."

"She did . . . ? When exactly?"

"I'm not sure, but you should call her."

"I will, thanks. Is she okay?"

"Oh, yeah, really good. She travels all over the world, you know, for her travel agency."

"Wow." Caroline, with severe colitis, had spent most of her youth either sick at home or in the hospital. She was the cousin most often absent from Sunday dinners and seders and picnics on the city beaches of Lake Michigan. After we moved to Texas, when I was eight, we kept hearing how ill Caroline was much of the time, and my parents phoned often to get reports.

"Bobs." I realized that for a moment I hadn't been listening.

"Yes, Jim, sorry."

"Haven't you had someone look at you constantly?"

"Jimmy, I have, really, all these years I've had every test invented." (Except a checkup, when I really knew something might be wrong. But I was too ashamed to admit that.)

"And?"

"I was always told I was just dandy. Not to worry. So in the last few years I saw things happening, but I thought it was a fissure . . ."

"And you ignored it?"

"I'm telling you, they told me it was hemorrhoids or a fissure or nerves." That much had been true.

"Barbara, our own grandmother had colon cancer."

"I'm just beginning to realize it," I said.

"Grandpa's brothers did too. So did Grandma with the White Hair . . ."

"Oh, Jimmy, remember how she never opened her windows, and her apartment always smelled of pot roast and old house plants?"

"I do, I do," he said, "she was a character, wasn't she? But she was our great-grandfather's *second* wife, and this is how far it goes back—they had a daughter, Sadie, and Sadie had twins, and they both got it."

"Dear God, the genes are coming from every direction," I said.

"And there was Grandpa's first cousin, Byron, and his father, Franklin, in Milwaukee."

I was having trouble listening to this, admitting it. Where had I been?

"And no one survived?" I asked.

"No, Bobs. *They all died.*"

"That's good news."

"Sorry, sorry." He paused for a moment. "I'm just worried about you, we all love you, we were kind of frantic when we heard you had already had the operation. I don't mean to upset you."

"Of course not." My vodka was gone. I got up to get ice and the bottle out of the freezer.

"But I just can't believe you didn't know all this. One of the uncles, I can't remember who, just made himself die. He couldn't cope with the bag anymore, and . . ."

That did it. I crashed against the wall in total defeat. Jay made a hand motion to end the phone call. He had an inkling what I was hearing, and he wanted it to stop.

"Jim dear, I must go. Things are burning on the stove." A blatant lie, but my stupidity about our family history was stunning me. I needed time to absorb all this, to stop talking for a while.

"Okay, okay. But first, please tell me how you're feeling." His concern was spoken in almost a whisper. Clearly distraught, he was trying to cover it with what he thought was chatty news. He really was so sweet, I couldn't be angry.

"Actually I feel fine, just discomfort from the stitches."

"Oh, you'll be healthy as ever. Just please take care of yourself."

"I will, thank you. How's Joan?"

"Oh, you know, the best and the most beautiful." He wasn't just making that up. His wife was a marvel: steadfast, full of humor, and utterly lovely.

"And the kids?"

"Oh, great. Allen's practice in Nevada is booming. Everybody's having babies. Grandchildren everywhere."

"Wonderful. Please give them all my love."

"I will. Now hang in there. We love you."

"Thanks, dear. I love you too."

I hung up and took a gulp of vodka, then walked into the den. I repeated much of the conversation to Jay, but my face was jerking around, and my eyes were anything but dry.

Jay said, "Barb, you know they must all be very anxious about you." He was trying to read his newspaper.

"I know. How many cousins take care of each other the way we do?"

"Absolutely none. Thank God." Back to the paper.

We both nodded ruefully. I sat down. "Jay, no one has survived."

"Honey, that was fifty, sixty years ago. The last one, your Uncle Burt, died in 1958. That's forty years. Procedures are much more advanced now," he said, clearly disappointed that he had to give up the reading.

"I know, but . . ."

"Look, your prognosis is excellent, and you should put this aside for an hour or two, do something you enjoy, something that keeps you busy. How about dinner? What can I do? Set the table?"

"You're indicating that you may be a little hungry?" I asked, rising from the sofa.

"I guess so," he said. "I'm also saying that you can't allow yourself a setback. You've got to push forward."

"I'll try, Jay."

"Good. Now what should I do?"

"Put trivets out, please, and um-m-m . . . open some red wine?"

"It's done. What else?"

"Take out the garbage and empty the dishwasher."

He walked over and put his arms around me. "And after I sweep the hearth, may I go to the ball?"

"Yes, Cinderella," I said.

He hugged me and headed into the kitchen. I followed behind him and began to cut vegetables for the salad.

Life barrels on.

CHAPTER 20

The Call to Caroline

I called Caroline Coen the next day at her home, a suburb of Chicago. She had already heard some of the story. Her no-nonsense, warm personality came leaping through the phone.

"Oh, Barbara, listen, you are going to be just dandy. This operation will open up a whole new life for you."

"It will?"

"You know how sick I was all my life."

"I do."

"Well, let me tell you. I have this little pouch now. I can do anything, go anywhere, and for the first time in my life, I can eat whatever I like. Of course I've gained twenty disgusting pounds, but I'll take care of that eventually."

"Caroline, did you have cancer?"

"Good heavens, no, but my gut was probably headed there. I had the ileostomy as an elective operation."

"Elective?" She had done this of her own free will? "And it's an ileostomy?"

"Sure, I had ulcerative colitis. An ileostomy takes care of that. The opening is into the small intestine, the small bowel. I don't have a rectum."

"I don't either."

"And I don't have a colon," she added.

"Well, I still have that," I said.

And then we started to giggle. This conversation was

unbelievable. It was as if we were talking about kitchen appliances.

"Do you know how many of our family have had some kind of bowel disorder, Barbara?"

"Jimmy clued me in," I said.

"We made an impromptu list not too long ago," she said, "and it was kind of shocking."

I sat up straight in my chair. "Did you keep a copy?"

"No, and I really should have."

"Why did you finally have the surgery?" I asked.

"Oh, Barbara, I was just finished with being in pain all the time, sitting on the aisle seat in the movie theater in case my stomach acted up. It finally got so bad that the doctor suggested I do it. So I did. It's just great. Unfortunately, there was a little trouble with the stoma, and I had to go back in."

"Oh, no."

"Yeah, that was no fun, but they fixed it, and I'm just fine." In the background I could hear another phone ring and someone calling, "Mom, are you here?"

"I can't tell you how helpful this is," I said.

"Well, I hope so. You've had problems for a long time?"

"Yes. For years. Constipation, fissures, you know."

"Do I ever."

"Then the last year, bleeding, all that," I said, with embarrassment. "I just kept it secret."

"Yeah, I understand," she sighed. "It's such a drag, such a private thing."

"Do you irrigate, Caroline?" It was a very personal question, but we were two people sharing an experience now, and I knew I could ask her anything.

"Oh, no. You can't with an ileostomy, it's just a constant thing. I change the pouch, big deal. I don't spend any more time in the bathroom than anyone else and go on my merry way. Dick and I are traveling all over the place, I don't have to worry about cramping or accidents or discomfort after all those years of being restricted and miserable."

"I gather your travel business is good," I said. "That's wonderful."

"It's really doing well, thanks for asking." Her deep Midwestern voice sounded pleased. "One of these days the four of us have got to do New Orleans. Remember that trip we were going to take?"

"I do," I answered. "I got a movie or something, what happened?"

"Oh, one of those things. In my line of work I'm prepared for anything."

"And the kids?" I asked.

"They all live out here," she said, "grandchildren, the whole shebang."

"Here's the big question," I said, but I knew it would be just another ordinary question for Caroline, who like her parents, Art and Hazel, always said whatever was on her mind, with no subterfuge or hidden agenda. "What about your sexual life?"

"Oh, gosh, it's fine. Just as before."

That was immensely reassuring news. "But I'm going to be pretty ashamed to show anyone this result, won't I, Caroline?"

"Well, don't. Why should you? Dick's never seen mine. It's just there. It doesn't change anything. The nice little bag covers it, no one has to think about it. You'll see, Barbara, things will be better than before."

"I hope so."

Her laugh was full of delight. "You have to believe me. I've just started to really live since this operation. Oh, and one more thing: When you dispose of the pouch, think 'tin foil.'"

"Oh, you wrap it in that?"

"Sure, I carry some with me. The foil really makes it secure, easier to throw away."

"Thanks for the tip," I said. "By the way, have you been to any ostomy support groups?"

"Yes, a couple here in Chicago, and they were helpful; but

I really didn't feel the need to continue. I did, however, join the United Ostomy Association . . ."

A pang of guilt gripped my heart. "I must do that," I said. "I've been so recalcitrant about sending a check."

"You've really got to. Just think how your donations can help other people, even if you don't need the assistance yourself. They do wonderful things."

"I'll do it immediately."

"Listen, I'm here any time you need me," Caroline said. "Call me day or night."

"I will. Thank you so much. Give my love to Dick and all your kids."

When I hung up the phone I knew that I had another ally. My own flesh and blood, a cousin I had always admired and loved, had experienced surgery, although hers was slightly different from mine. She was flying high, jubilant about her health, and most movingly, she had shared her absolute certainty that, for me, a life of better quality lay ahead.

In the early 1900s her grandmother, Caroline Lapine, had died, and my grandparents raised the Lapine children along with their own three kids: two adults and seven children in four crowded, hectic rooms on the South Side of Chicago.

Those seven children became like brothers and sisters, cherishing one another, arguing as families do, raising *their* children, my generation, like siblings. Through the years, we had all remained close; and here, today, was that thread of history and affection weaving its way from Poland-Germany to Canada to Wisconsin, then from Chicago, to us, two second cousins living in far-apart cities.

Caroline became over time my role model, my symbol of encouragement. Without her I would never have survived the problems that lay ahead, although, when we first spoke I had no idea what they were to be. Her good cheer, her joyous attitude toward her new life, and her touching concern for me thrust me forward in the determination to survive.

CHAPTER 21

A Kelly Checkup

Around May 21, I didn't seem to be healing. The black stitches, crisscrossed around the stoma like a quilted design, were leathery-looking and inflamed. Weren't they supposed to dissolve?

It became difficult to walk, particularly up and down stairs because the skin felt as if it were being clawed by cats. I really hate cats, and it was a nasty analogy that kept grabbing at me (a pun *intended*).

I called Terry Haus at the hospital. "Oh, Barbara, that pulling is pretty routine," she said. "When's your next appointment with Dr. Kelly? He'll explain it all."

"Not for another week or so, Terry, and I don't think I can wait. I can't do anything!"

"Well, call up and say you have to see him. I'll meet you there."

Two days later Dr. Kelly and Terry were peering at the bomb site, which was how I now thought of this operation. The summer sun flooded the examining room, backlighting Terry's hair. Dr. Kelly's white coat crackled as he wheeled over on his metal stool.

"Don't you think those stitches should come out?" asked Terry, treading a careful verbal track so that Dr. Kelly would not feel he was being usurped.

"Absolutely not. These stitches will dissolve. You'll just have to put up with a little nuisance, Barbara. In a week they'll be gone."

"But Dr. Kelly, every move is a pull or a stab," I said. "Can't we take just a few out so that I can at least walk on the street and not hobble like an injured war veteran?"

A peculiar look wrinkled his face. Had I overstepped my boundaries? "Look," he said, "I put these stitches in, and I know what they will do. Now let's wait a few days and see if they don't dissolve. That's what they're supposed to do, and that's what they'll do."

Terry glanced quickly at me and lowered her head as she covered me with the paper robe. "Okay, whatever you say," she said, plainly frustrated. "Could she have some kind of mild painkiller? I'll give her some cream to apply to the stoma."

Dr. Kelly stood up. "That sounds good, Terry. I'll write out a prescription, you give her the cream. Whatever helps," he said. "Barbara, I'll see you in a week or so."

He whipped around and was out the door in a second. Not a "good-bye" or "call me anytime" or "hope you feel better."

A week later, bent over like the witch in Hansel and Gretel and clutching the doorknob, I limped into the examining room and collapsed onto the table. The pain was now so cutting and incessant that I was having trouble even drawing a deep breath.

"Well, those stitches are still there, aren't they?" he said, as if he were conducting a class in surgical procedure.

Terry, who was holding my hand, said, "Dr. Kelly, can't you please take them out now? Haven't they been in too long? They're so inflamed."

"Yes, that's interesting," he said. "I just don't understand why they haven't dissolved. Maybe we should wait a few more days."

"No," I said. "Dr. Mears says I can't start the radiation until I've healed. I have visions of the tumor spreading all over the place."

"There's just a slight irregularity here, that's all," he said, squinting again at the bumpy, distorted area.

Terry smiled, soft-pedaling her concern into the touchy atmosphere. "Dr. Kelly, don't you think . . ."

"All right," he said. After a long pause, "I'll go get some instruments." And he left the room.

I raised myself on one elbow. "What is it with him, Terry? Why do I feel as if he doesn't want to help me?"

"I don't know that he doesn't, Barbara."

"Tell me something. Isn't this stoma too big? Am I always going to have this aperture hanging from my body?"

Without looking in my direction, she said, "Barbara, I think we have to wait to see if it will retract. It is swollen, but I think it will go down. Try not to make any judgments now. Just get the stitches out—they really must come out—and see what happens."

Dr. Kelly, instruments in hand, reentered the room. He removed the black, stubborn stitches. They certainly had not dissolved: Each time he snipped one out, I could feel the sting and then the relaxing of the flesh that had been crunched up by the thread.

"I feel better already," I said. "Thank you, Dr. Kelly." What I had really wanted to say was, "Why didn't we do this last week?" But again it was the "white coat" syndrome: The doctor knows best, doesn't he?

Another doctor might have asked all kinds of questions in a calm, helpful manner. He or she might have talked to me about the various ways to alleviate the pain and the prospects for the next few days.

Terry and I parted at the Broadway entrance of the hospital. Many people in wheelchairs, accompanied by hovering, exhausted relatives, were waiting there for Ambulettes to take them home. Radiation patients, on their way to the lab downstairs, swung through the revolving doors, their heads wrapped in scarves or covered by baseball caps.

Terry and I embraced. I held on to her for a few minutes. As I walked toward the subway at 168th Street, I took my first full steps in weeks. There was only a shadow of pain, and I could at last stand up straight. I walked down the steps and onto the elevator leading to the Seventh Avenue subway. I couldn't believe it. I was not clutching my belly nor breathing in short, torturous gasps. A miracle.

At least for now.

CHAPTER 22

Radiation-Chemo

This could be called the Chemotherapy-Radiation Scenario. I was to begin radiation and chemo at the same time: twenty-four hours on a chemo drip and a daily dose of radiation at Columbia Presbyterian Hospital. What fun.

The drug prescribed was 5-fluorouracil, which is an antimetabolic (a chemical, of course) that mimics one of the building blocks of DNA. The goal, Dr. Mears had told me, is to interfere with the process of DNA synthesis, to "screw it up" and keep the cell from dividing and continuing its deadly proliferation. The 5-fluorouracil, they think, improves the effectiveness of the radiation, although no one is really sure how it all works.

"You're not sure?" I practically screeched.

Dr. Mears shrugged. "Look, a cell must make new chromosomes. If we can damage it before it divides, it may stop the cancer cells from multiplying. The theory is not fully understood, but it's what we have now. It's why, if people knew about cell mechanism, they wouldn't resort to apricot pits and weird injections, although . . . ," he paused, "we do think now that green tea might halt the growth of tumors."

"So you never know for sure?"

"Well, we keep trying."

Dr. Mears had arranged for a room in a part of the hospital donated by some rich patient many years ago. A full entertainment system had been built into the deco-styled wood paneling: VCR, a large-screen TV, a cassette player, radio, and all the accompanying equipment unable to be used by a mechanical failure like me.

Only when Jane came to visit could she do her magic shenanigans so that we could actually see a movie or hear a concerto. For hours she would sit with me as we watched rented films or previously taped television shows, and we gossiped, although occasionally I would doze for a few hazy minutes in this 1930s-like room where Myrna Loy would have felt totally at ease.

Sometimes she seemed to drift away, out of the room, with her own thoughts. "Janie, are you worried about me?" I asked one day. "Because I honestly think I'm going to be fine, I just want you to know that."

"Oh, I agree. After the doctor came out of the operating room and said you were okay, I really never worried again."

"But sometimes you don't speak for long moments."

"Well, Mom, we've all been through a lot in the last month, and I've made two trips back and forth, so I guess I'm just tired. And, excuse me, but I have my own life too."

"I know, darling."

"Well, I'll tell you now that once I was really upset," she said as she poured us both some ice water. "Just after I went back to L.A., after you were out of the hospital, I was seeing Dr. Green."

"The psychologist?" I asked.

"Yes, Juliette Green, and I remember one day I was driving to therapy, I was flipping around on the dial, and there was a song on the radio about a mother and daughter, and the mother—throughout the daughter's life—every time she loses a best friend or loses a husband . . ."

"The daughter loses?" I asked.

"Yes, the daughter. And the mother is always there for her. And the mother keeps telling the daughter all through the song, I can't remember the lyrics right now, but that 'time heals all, you'll get over this, life is always changing, we have to say good-bye'; and at the end of the song the mother is dying and the daughter is at her bedside, and of course I started weeping."

"Well, of course," I said, about to weep myself. "What's it called?"

"I don't know. It's a station I never listen to," Jane said, as she drew her small leather journal out of her knapsack. "Oh, here it is . . . yes, May 21, in the car."

"How long did you cry, Jane?"

"Oh, not very long. I was almost at therapy."

We both laughed.

Wherever I went, the IV accompanied me on its shaky metal pole. To the bathroom, to the window, while I slept, on a walk down the hall with Jay or Jane, to teatime in the solarium every afternoon.

But no visitors, even though more and more people knew what had happened. I did accept phone calls now, and some friends called often. Others sent flowers, and I must say they were welcomed. Occasionally I would call back, but something told me that privacy and quiet were the things that would make me well. And I refused to be a burden to my friends.

When an attendant came to wheel me through the labyrinth of hospital corridors, I was temporarily unattached from the IV bottle. A relief, not to have it wavering over my shoulder all the time. Then down to the radiation lab in another building, the Babies Hospital, where, under blankets on the gurney, I would wait my turn.

Surrounding me were people who appeared to be much sicker than I. Barely awake, they looked as if they had ceased to struggle, as if they were undergoing a ritual that would not provide them much more of life. Sometimes it seemed as if we were all forgotten. Activities swirled around us, but we lay for very long periods with no one speaking or bringing us up to date on the schedule. The other patients didn't seem to care, and that horrified me.

I did care and I did want to know and I didn't feel sick (that came later) and I kept telling myself that I was not as ill as they, that I refused to give up, that I wanted my radiation zap, and then I wanted to go back to my glamorous room and have tea.

Eventually I would get my few seconds of glory beneath the giant machine, and I would wait again until someone came to take me back to the other building. That was acceptable. Even though I had to wait, I felt that one more step had been taken toward recovery. It was to be five days of this dual treatment. I hated it, but I also welcomed it. I was a warrior.

Intensive doses of 5-fluorouracil give you unbelievable mouth sores, and about the third day, the combination of the chemo and radiation makes you feel like a radio on FM and AM tuning at the same time. Dr. Mears had warned me that the sores might develop, so I had Jay bring to the hospital my Water Pik, ten toothbrushes, toothpaste, mouthwash, and dental floss—waxed and unwaxed, plain, cinnamon-flavored.

After every meal I used all of these things, assiduously scrubbing, washing, rinsing, flossing. Forget it. I got gruesome mouth sores the minute I returned home, and they lasted for about a week. Then they were gone.

Dr. Mears visited every day. He'd sit in one of the chairs, cross his long legs, and settle down for an unhurried exchange. Once more I noticed that he seemed not rushed, as if he could spend this hour with me and really enjoy it. This is called Bedside Manner. It is also called Humanity. We talked of his son's soccer meets, of bringing up kids, of the latest political events, and of the cancer.

I was doing well, he said, but I still had the whole program of radiation ahead, seven and a half weeks of almost-daily treatment. "For that time you'll be off the chemo."

"But I started it already. Why stop now?"

He shook his head. "It's just the way we do it," he said. "We give you a jump-start, then withhold the chemo until the radiation is complete."

"Is this what most rectal cancer patients get, this course of treatment?"

"Yes," he said. "It's quite usual. Nothing fancy."

He handed me a prescription for the mouth sores. "And when you begin your weekly sessions, I'll also be giving you some pills to take every other week."

"Called what?" I asked, making a face.

"Ergamisol. It's a fairly tough drug."

"I see," I said.

"Some people don't react at all. This radiation is a powerful influence, you know. It attacks the cell nucleus, and it's preventive, it eliminates worry."

"And the chemo too?"

"Also preventive. It's a light dose. It's also the usual procedure for your kind of tumor. You may not have any side effects."

"But we can't be sure?" I asked.

"No, we can't be sure," he said, kindly, trying to soften the blow.

A stiffness suddenly attacked my neck. I couldn't move. I felt besieged. "Dr. Mears, tell me the truth, do you think I'll get through this?"

A truly serious look passed across his face. "I think your progress is amazing. Part of recovery, you know, is the spirit of the patient, the will to live. Whatever you're doing, just keep it up, okay?"

"Okay," I said. If he believed in me, surely I could beat this rap.

I just had to.

CHAPTER 23

The Lady on the Bus

JUNE 30, 1994

There were bananas, lettuce, asparagus, and artichokes in my shopping bag as I walked home from the market, my first "wifely chores" since the five-day double dose of chemotherapy and radiation. I bought tissue paper at the local economy store—what a joy, to be doing a real thing in the real world, away from hospitals and doctors. I counted out the change, then grabbed two rolls of Life Savers.

"That'll be sixty-five cents more," said the cashier.

"Gladly," I said, thrilled to be standing there, the sun struggling through the spotted windows, bits of trash over the floor. It was all simply wonderful.

I ordered a case of wine from Mike, our local wine merchant, who said, "Welcome! Where have you been? Off doing a movie or something?"

"No, I was just vacationing." (Ha!)

He proceeded to tell me a long story about his wife's recent entry into medical school. A very long story. I relished every moment of it. Asking him many questions, I finally realized forty-five minutes had passed. Ordinarily I would have long ago rushed away to the next unimportant, benign activity, but today I was fascinated by the conversation and delighted by the bins of wine with their large white price signs: "Best of the newest California Pinot Noir." Yes, yes, I would take two cases, and I would adore any narrative, any bit of news, even the local panhandler who dizzily held out his hand as I left the store.

I was an alive person on 72nd Street, Zip Code 10023.

The sun warmed my back, so I opened my jacket. The breeze lifted my hair as I walked with slightly tentative, sneakered steps. Overhead the clouds moved in summertime, scuddery shapes from the Hudson River toward Fire Island.

Oh joy, oh wonder, oh mystical Fire Island, my heart's residence, my solace, my peaceful place.

I once asked my therapist friend Jeffrey Kramer, "Why am I so in love with Saltaire? It's just like Corpus Christi—on the water, sailboats, cottages, the white beach. Our little house is exactly like the one I grew up in. And my life at home was so hideous, you know that. What makes being at the beach so emotional for me?"

"Because this time you're going to make it right," he replied.

We'd soon be going to Saltaire for weekends. I'd have to do the seven or more weeks of radiation from Monday to Friday. Yet there was still a kind of stretching, pulling pain, and the lumpy shape of the new opening could clearly be seen beneath any fitted garment. Wasn't it supposed to conform to my body? I thought by now the edema was supposed to subside.

In our elevator I moved quickly into the corner, put down the shopping bags. Too many people crowded in after me, and I extended my arms as if to ward off an enemy. I didn't want anyone too close, I was afraid of being bumped, the colostomy being hit. The afternoon had been so freeing and happy, and suddenly, in a moment, I was a little old lady, the kind who used to make me impatient and resentful. Now I was one of them!

"Jay, I'm turning into a crone. I'm a little old lady." I cried, as he came home from rehearsal. "I'm scared of human contact."

"Well, right now you are. Of course. Stay calm, Barbara, why do you expect so much of yourself?" He put down his shoulder bag. "Come on, I'm taking you out for dinner."

The first time in an enclosed, public place? What if everyone could see that I was carrying around this new, projecting, raw attachment? What if the pouch broke, and the entire restaurant would view this overflowing, smelly, bent-over woman rushing to the ladies' room with her supplies in hand?

"So if you have an accident, you have an accident," Jay said. "Big deal. How many other people in concert halls and theaters and restaurants probably have had the same operation? Darling, I hate to say this, but you are not that important, and you are not alone in this thing."

That's telling the little old lady.

We went to a Spanish restaurant in Greenwich Village where we had had one of our first dates in 1964. It was still the same: candles and pitchers of sangria, baskets of addicting bread, and checked tablecloths. Tonight we had paella and red wine and salad. It was almost romantic, except that I was slightly tense, and the pouch seemed to be puffing out. The pressure was uncomfortable, so I shifted often on the cushioned booth.

As Jay was paying the check, I went into the ladies' room to see what was happening. Yes, it was just air, but the pouch was hugely blown up and unbearably tight. I took off one of my earrings and with the post made a tiny hole. The pouch sighed with relief and relaxed a little. Wasn't I smart to think of that? I was proud of my inventiveness.

Back on Seventh Avenue Jay said, "Shall we go into the chess place and have a game, the way we used to?"

We gazed into the chess parlor where, twenty-five years ago, we had spent a few evenings laughing and courting and drinking tepid coffee. I could never beat Jay, even though I was a fair player. And I couldn't have cared less. I had just been waiting until we could go back to my sublet apartment, take a long, warm bath together, and make love.

"No, forgive me, honey, I think I've had enough. Would you mind taking me home?"

"Shall we get a cab?"

"No, no, a bus is fine. I need to get used to people." We boarded a Number 7 bus. Jay put his arm around me, as if to protect me from a falling passenger or a jolt or a sudden stop.

As we progressed uptown, I began to enjoy the ride, but the pouch seemed to be doing a little rumba under my clothes, and then a huge, solid expulsion entered it from my body. Oh, dear. Why couldn't it wait until we got home? Well, it'd be okay, wouldn't it? I mean the pouch would take care of it. No one would know.

Gradually a really vile smell came up from my belly. I mean, a violently awful, terrible, embarrassing, traumatic, ghastly smell. I actually wanted to die, to melt into the atmosphere, to disappear. No one told me that I would ever experience such humiliation. I was subhuman, a leper, something to be thrown out.

I drew my coat around me tightly. Why was this happening? The odor became worse, and the woman next to me began to sniff and look under her feet. Oh, my God. She thought a dog had been there, or there must be garbage on the floor.

I flattened my arms across the coat. The woman became more frantic in her search. She rose and looked at her seat, then sat back down again. I was paralyzed. I couldn't move. If I moved, she'd know it was my fault. Staring straight ahead, I tried to pretend that absolutely nothing was happening. Jay was sleeping against my shoulder. He has slept through a California earthquake and a two-and-a-half-hour broadcast of the Metropolitan Opera, so I wasn't surprised that he was oblivious of this unspeakable crisis.

The woman began to whimper as if she were caught in the throes of a demonic, whirling draft, but she didn't move either. It was as if we were bound together by a nightmare neither of us was willing to acknowledge or believe.

She took out a tissue and looked at the bottom of her shoes.

Had she stepped in something? She looked up at the air vents and tried to open a window. A man tried to help her, but it was bolted shut. She sat down again, rigid, bewildered.

And now she was getting angry.

Finally she turned and looked straight at me, her eyes wide, full of furious realization. She wanted to kill me. And I didn't blame her. I stared back in horror. I wanted to say, "No, you are not crazy and it is me and I've just had cancer and a colostomy and I don't know how to handle it and please accept my apology." But my lips were zippered, my neck stiff. I desperately wanted to face the moment, to be honest, to take her out of her misery, but I couldn't do it.

A minute later we reached 72nd Street, and I rushed to the door, leaving her with her hand across her mouth and nose, her face perspiring. Poor soul. I had nearly done her in.

It was of course the hole I had punched in the pouch. You're not supposed to do that: It lets the smell out. And I was so stupid, such a novice, that only now did I understand the consequences of what I'd done. A hole in the pouch is a no-no. An absolute, irrevocable, unrelenting no-no.

I told Jay what had happened as we walked home. He could smell me now.

"Wow!" He started to laugh. "You are a little fragrant."

"Oh, sorry, I'm so sorry." I moved toward the curb. "But Jay, this is tragic . . . that poor woman," I said.

"Oh, she's just fine. It should be the worst thing that ever happens to her. Lighten up, for chrissakes, Barbara." He was still laughing.

"Do you think she'll go home and have chocolate cake and milk, now or ever again?" I asked.

"Yes, and in twenty minutes she'll forget all about it. She'll dine out on that story for months."

I wondered if I could ever tell the same story, if I'd have the courage or the humor to do it. Truthfully, it had been funny, horrific, and bizarre. And that's the moment when I decided, in a flash, to write this book.

CHAPTER 24

Radiation

The subway ride from West 72nd Street and Broadway to Columbia Presbyterian Hospital at 168th Street is easy. The trains come often, and in the middle of the morning they are uncrowded. Sometimes I'd go up on the C or B train that stops at Central Park West and 72nd Street, but those trains are infrequent, and the empty platform often echoes with all the brutal stories on the nightly six o'clock news.

Seven and a half to eight weeks of radiation had been prescribed. That meant every day, except for weekends. ("We don't treat cancer on Saturdays and Sundays," Dr. Mears had said, with an ironic smile.) That meant staying in the city all week and leaving for Fire Island on Friday afternoon.

Beginning on June 16, 1994, I rode the subway every day. I entered at the Babies Hospital entrance and took the elevator down to the basement radiation clinic, where I presented my blue-cased plastic identification card.

I was on the computer, a statistic, one of the thousands of people who arrive here ill and hope to leave cured: a bald Dominican child accompanied by his entire family, elderly white couples holding hands, a lone worker in dusty blue jeans, an obese college professor who talks always of going on a diet, a willowy black woman wearing a Cartier bracelet and carrying an Hermés bag.

And me. Usually in pants or a summer skirt (it was getting very warm in New York) with my current reading material, my glasses, my straw bag. There was a coffee room I never went in because everyone there talked about his or her illness and treatment. Was I one of them? Of course not. I was having "preventive" radiation—it was to make sure that nothing would come back, no tumor or spot. I was really okay, wasn't I? I was thin but not emaciated like some of the patients brought down on gurneys from the hospital upstairs. I was walking, keeping house, riding the subway. I was just dandy. I could sit in the waiting room outside, read my book, make some phone calls, have my treatment, and get on with my life.

For the first few weeks I put on the prescribed gown, left my clothes and panties in a locker, and climbed up on the table. Dennis, the young, hip technician, was friendly and almost casual as he arranged my limbs and smoothed the gown under the giant telescopelike machine that would zap me. "We have to be precise," he said, "so that the radiation goes exactly to the target. We don't want to treat the wrong area, even by a hundredth of an inch."

I pulled the gown tight around me. "Dennis, this pouch of mine is full, I want you to know that."

"It doesn't matter at all." He adjusted the monster eye above me a fraction of an inch as he positioned my hips a breath to the left. "I've seen everything, much worse than that by about a hundred miles."

"But it's embarrassing," I said, still clutching the gown. "I can't irrigate yet." I had never before said that word to a stranger.

"Oh, sure, that takes time, but you'll get there. Now let's open the robe so I can see the target."

Looking in the other direction, I exposed the bag, and it was indeed full. Drat. This was a low, low point. On the outside of my body, my insides were clearly visible. Why didn't I just walk around naked all the time and get it over with?

He gently pressed my right shoulder closer to the table and once more placed both hands on my hips and rolled me slightly to the left—like a slab of salmon at Zabar's as the fish man plops it down on the cutting board.

"But Dennis, I never know what's going to happen with this damned pouch."

"Forget it. We're prepared for everything here." He smiled, his handsome face dimpling, his wavy black hair falling over his forehead. "When is *Scarlett* going to be on?"

We'd chat for a minute or two, then he'd leave, the thick iron door closing behind him as I stared up into the machine, the room cold and silent. I was totally exposed from the waist down.

There would be a brief hum and a click as the radiation zeroed in on the infinitesimal black tattoo on my right hip.

Back came Dennis to reposition the machine over the tattoo on my left hip. Once more he would carefully move my body: one inch to the left, the arm up just so, the other arm down, the knee turned in. When satisfied, he would leave again, the door wheezing shut, the machine making its solitary noise in the cell-like room.

This procedure would be repeated until all the other little crosslike tattoos had been exposed—all the places in the lower part of my body that might harbor another tumor: the pubis area, the vagina, the buttocks. (What if it got into my vagina? I'd give up. I wouldn't let them do anything else. I'd just ask for pills and get out.)

Aaron had said, "Mom, are you 'imaging'? Don't waste time when you're lying there. Imagine the exact spot where you're being zapped and *will* it to work." So that's what I did, even though (it's hard to believe) I eventually became so comfortable and so focused from the imaging that I slept or dozed most of the time; Dennis would have to whisper, "We're done."

He helped me sit up, close the gown, and lower myself to the floor. "Dennis, now that you've seen my entire body in its total, uncontrolled state, don't you think you should call me Barbara?"

He laughed. "I'll try, but I don't think I can do that."

After a few weeks I asked him, "Do I have to put on that gown? Can't I just skip the locker room and come right here? I could take off my clothing and hop up on the table."

I could tell from his face that I'd be breaking the rules. He looked around, ducked his head, and said softly, "Why not? Just come back to this area in your clothes, but don't broadcast it to everyone."

From then on I whipped off my trousers and underwear, climbed up on the table, and we proceeded. If I was wearing a skirt, I just slipped off my panties, hiked up the material, and lay down. Sometimes the pouch was flat, sometimes full, and Dennis would adjust it slightly—actually move it around so that the rays could hit their destination. It became one of the givens of the situation: The pouch was a player. As soon as we were finished he and one of his assistants would help me off the table, I'd dress in a nanosecond, and off I'd go, back into the subway, off on 72nd Street, and home to our apartment.

Radiation is cumulative. It seemed so easy at first, although after a few weeks I did notice a slowing down of everything I did, as if I were floating or dreaming. Tasks took longer to accomplish; crossing the street seemed like fording a swiftly flowing stream. Knowing I should shop for vegetables, I'd look at the Fairway crowds, wave to Heshie Hochman, turn around, and go haltingly home, my feet, seemingly unattached to my legs, flapping on the sidewalk.

As the radiation began to tunnel through tissue, I began to get wildly sore, red, irritated. My labial area began to burn and peel; so did the lower part of my buttocks—almost like a severe diaper rash—and the inside of my thighs. The sympathetic, smiling nurses would take me into a treatment room and rub soothing salves and lotions over all the areas. I was told to take sitz baths at home. Sometimes I spent two or three hours a day immersed in water, in Manhattan and on Fire Island over the weekends.

"Why is Barbara in the tub all the time?" asked a friend as Jay met her at the door of our house.

"Oh, she's got a bad heat rash on her tush," Jay said. "Or else she doesn't want to make dinner, who knows?"

Almost no one in Saltaire had any idea that I was ill. I was not ready to be viewed as a "poor soul," and I didn't want to be, above all, a bore, always talking about my white cell count, my treatments, my progress, my doctors. I had seen too much of that. It was a role I didn't want to play in a production that interested me not at all.

Many cancer patients need to talk about their illnesses, their treatments, what the doctor said, what he or she didn't say, how they're feeling, what the latest tests disclose, and I believe that's therapeutic for them. I honor their need to communicate with friends and family about their states of mind and health.

I see that other people, in the very act of talking, bring themselves back into the world. They are alive, they're ambulatory, they can work, but they need to share this terrible thing they are going through, and the assurance and sympathy they receive must help to make them well. But it was simply not my way.

Now, years later, people are telling me that they didn't know how I could have kept such secrets. They had played tennis with me, attended village meetings, eaten dinner at our house, even come to a play I had done much later (while I was still in chemotherapy). But remaining private was, I believed, my way of getting well.

During my solitary hours in the tub, I got a lot of reading done, but the irritations were very, very painful. Twice, Dr. Hayes, the supervising physician, halted the treatments for a while. "You're just too sore," she said. "Take a little rest and come back in two weeks."

It was a reprieve from hell. I could go to Fire Island and try to resume my life. I did swim a lot (the salt water was soothing) and play tennis, although a year later, when my game had improved wildly, I realized how badly I'd been playing: The radiation had slowed my reflexes and running ability. I couldn't understand how a ball could fly by me at the net and I didn't hold up my racquet to bounce it back. I was drifting in the air like protoplasm and wasn't aware of it at all. I just cursed my lack of ability and refused to play with anyone but close friends.

Chemotherapy was still ahead of me, but I felt guilty about not working for so long. After all, I had almost ceased contributing my share of a two-income family.

"Jay, are we going to be all right? I'm not earning anything except residuals" (payment for television shows done in the past). We were making breakfast at the beach, ducking out of each other's way as we buttered toast and poured coffee.

"You look exhausted," he said, handing me a glass of juice, "the way you did when Jane and Aaron were little and you were up all night."

"I *was* up all night. I'm worried about money. I mean, I know my medical bills are covered, but how about everything else . . . you know, the mortgage, all that stuff?"

"Barbara, you've worked for years." We carried the tray out to the deck. "Just 'chill out' now, as the kids used to say, and stop thinking about that. We're in good shape." We opened the umbrella and sat down at the table. "We're very lucky people, you know, to have as much as we do."

My money anxiety was almost alleviated that morning, although it always returned during my 3 A.M. waking times, when everything that ever drives me crazy comes zooming into my head like a squadron of air force fighter planes.

But during the day I was happy. I watered the flowers on the sunny deck, the thump of the ocean misting through the pine trees. We sat by the fire on cool nights. I painted furniture and took power walks with Letty and Bobbie. I played tennis. Jay and I made love again in our breeze-swept bedroom.

I clung, at first, to my side of the bed. "What if I don't remember how to do it?" I asked. "It's been almost three months."

"I may not remember either," he said, lying very still, as

though he, too, was afraid to begin. "We'll just start and see what happens. It must be like riding a bike—you never forget . . ."

". . . how," we both said together. It was one of our old, creaky jokes.

The moonlight glimmered onto the deck and into our window. It also glimmered on the beige plastic pouch (empty, thank God) resting upon my belly. I pulled the sheet over my left hip. "Jay, is this thing going to totally turn you off?"

"Barbara, I've told you, I couldn't care less. Besides, I really think it's kind of adorable." I laughed. We had put on the Beethoven Triple Concerto, the genius sound of Yo-Yo Ma drifting from the living room. Listening, we lay still and held hands, getting up the courage to begin. The electric fan whirred on the dresser.

There was a tentative kiss, a hand cupping my chin, then another hand on my buttocks, which were now just the covering of the departed rectum.

"Does this hurt?" he asked.

"No, not at all," I said. He drew me closer, and then suddenly a gust of heat, like a Texas garden in August, rose up between our bodies. I put my arms around his back. Oh, yes, I remembered this back, the way one side is more muscular than the other. There was the smell of his aftershave and the soft shag of his neck. Suddenly the barrier disappeared. We sighed into each other.

"I think we're riding this bicycle," said Jay. He kissed my ear.

We did just fine. I wept that it was still possible, that the sensations were still there. Afterward, Jay held me and wiped my eyes with a tissue. "You made so much noise," he said. "I was afraid the police would come."

"I wouldn't have cared," I said, still crying, still shaking, still thrilled.

"So now, Mrs. Harnick, would you like a glass of water?"

"Definitely," I said. Back to everyday life. Water, a bit of face cream, readjusting the bed linens. Wonderful.

Two years later, as we were making our bed together, I asked Jay what he was really thinking that night.

He looked as if I had just read his secret diary. "I was wondering how many more times we would be able to do this thing we've always had. I mean, making love." He looked at me across the bed. "I thought 'how much longer do we have together?' Mortality. It was the quickness of mortality that struck me."

A huge admission from someone like Jay, who hardly ever reveals his fears.

"But of course you didn't tell me," I said.

"Well, no. Certainly not at the moment we were beginning to make love. Anyway, you know I can never express my immediate thoughts. It's our really big problem, isn't it? You scream and cry and holler, and I repress almost everything."

"I'll say," I replied. I arranged two more pillows as he smoothed the quilt. "You actually thought I might die?"

"Barbara, how could I not? You had been in danger. You had just had major surgery and radiation. I have feelings. I am not a thing of stone."

I nodded. That's another of our corny sayings.

He started to put on his shirt as I sat down at my desk. "Another thing," he said, "I was also in total admiration of the way you had handled everything, the appliance problem and the irrigation, working with Terry to learn how to do it."

"You were thinking of all that on the very night . . . ?" I asked, turning in my chair.

"I thought about it almost every day," he said. "And I was aware that you were trying to shield me. You didn't want me to see the pouch, you still don't . . ."

"But you see it now when we make love or when I walk around without clothes."

"Yes, but you tried to cover it for a long time."

"Oh, I really didn't think about the pouch," I said, "but I've never shown you the actual opening."

"No, you haven't."

"Do you want to see it?"

"Yes, in a way I would." He began to walk out of the room and then turned back. That "here comes a joke" look flickered around his mouth. "I'm not exactly *eager* to see it, but in fact, I'm curious."

I laughed. "Would you like to make an appointment for the viewing?"

"Sure. How about tonight?"

"Okay," I said. "I'd show it to you now, but I've just done my irrigation thing, and I haven't even had a shower."

"I wouldn't care," he said, as he came closer and sat on the window seat.

"No, Jay, I can't. I've got to be really clean and fresh. You know it's one of my unshakable habits."

"Just the way you have to make the bed the minute your feet hit the floor in the morning?" he asked.

"Yes," I replied. "Call me silly."

"It's okay," he said. I swiveled back to the computer, but he didn't move. "And another thing I thought at that time . . ."

Wow! This man was talking! "Yes?" I asked.

"You were very busy protecting everyone, trying to keep the burden from us," he said, "so what you did and what you do, is to put more of it on yourself."

His tanned face and white hair were in beautiful contrast to his blue denim shirt and flowered tie. For the first time in many months, maybe years, he was telling me what his deepest feelings had been. He looked clear and open, almost as if releasing the truth had relaxed him, eased the lines of his face, straightened his shoulders.

"Maybe because my mother was always such a kvetch," I said, "always crying, sick, complaining. I just didn't want to be like her."

"Yes, honey, but you bend the other way. You do too much for people. You try to protect everyone, particularly me and the kids."

"But isn't friendship 'doing things' for people, helping them?"

160

"To a certain extent. But you go overboard." He stood and picked up his canvas shoulder bag. "You've got to get on with it, live your life, stop worrying about everyone else."

"Okay, I'll try. I'm grateful that you're telling me all this."

He waved. "Good-bye, hon. I'll pick up Jane at the airport and see you tonight."

I remained at my desk for a long time. I'd said all along that cancer had been bringing me odd, unexpected gifts. Today, this conversation with my husband had been one of them.

On July 27, 1994, the treatments were finally finished. The nurses and Dr. Hayes and Dennis bid me a fond farewell, and I was free, for a while. In three months I would have another visit and checkup with Dr. Mears, another CAT scan and blood tests. Before that, however, chemotherapy would begin. Amazingly, in less than two weeks all the irritation and sores were gone.

The little tattoos remain forever, purply-black, tiny and indelible, on my body. Occasionally I see one as I'm drying myself off after a shower, and it's always a surprise.

Most of the time I completely forget they are there.

CHAPTER 25

Irrigation Failure, Saltaire

SEPTEMBER 1994

Terry Haus was coming to Fire Island. This weekend was the Great Irrigation Teach-in. I was finally going to learn to regulate my elimination, to be a free soul, unleashed from worry, accidents, and discomfort.

The chemotherapy had begun on August 31, and although I would have reported to the hospital in New York every Thursday, our cherished Saltaire doctor, "Dr. Bob" Furey, had arranged for me to receive the treatment in his office. This saved me from a weekly trip on the ferry, the train, and the subway, which was a pure blessing.

The Ergamisol pills, taken every other week on Monday, Tuesday, and Wednesday, were beginning to feel like poison, but so far I had been able to get through it.

The stoma had lost its redness, but it seemed to sit on my body like a small balloon from outer space, a piece of intestine dangling on my belly. I still thought, however, that this was the nature of all colostomies: protruding, painful, hard to manage.

On a sparkling Saturday morning Terry alighted from the ferry with a bag of groceries and a bottle of wine. We loaded her belongings into our little red wagon and walked slowly toward our house. Her knees seemed better than usual, but I worried about the fairly long distance.

"No, forget it. I walk more than this at the hospital. I'm just so thrilled to be here," she said. "Look at those flowers. Isn't the sky beautiful? Can we spend the afternoon on the beach?"

We talked under the umbrella at the ocean after lunch. We dozed and laughed. She told me about her latest beau, an old flame she had met long ago in Israel.

"He still calls." She gradually settled into the beach chair. "But the perfect time has passed, you know?"

"But you liked him so much in the dear, dead days beyond," I said.

"The really dear, dead days, Barbara." She pulled a towel around her legs as the beach darkened and grew cool. "But I've got my patients, and he lives a million miles away. How can I manage all that?"

"Oh, Terry, you're just not that interested. 'Mr. Right' is still around the corner."

"Oh, yeah?" She laughed and actually slapped her knee. "Well, we'll see!"

We wound a sandy trail back to the house. After showers and a long drink on the deck, we all made dinner in our cozy, cramped kitchen. We ate by the fireplace, the candles flickering on the white walls and the old, blue-stained rafters.

The next morning she announced that the time had come. Gathering all the irrigation equipment, we went into the bathroom.

I placed the long plastic sleeve around my waist and secured it with the mesh belt. I sat down on the toilet. By now it seemed nothing at all. I could sit naked, unnaked, spread-eagled, on my side, on my back in front of anyone. Bring in the cameras, bring in the doctors, gather the statistic-makers. I was imperturbable.

She filled the irrigation bag with warm water, then hung it by a coat hanger to a hook in the door about eight inches above my head.

"Now we're going to insert this tip into the opening, through the top of the sleeve," she said. "First, you know, we have to let the water run out a little to get rid of the bubbles. Goodness, you're still too thin. Breathe in a bit, Barbara, sit up straight, please."

I held my breath and pulled up my torso as high as I could. Terry peered through the top of the sleeve.

"Hm-m-m, what's this?"

"What's what?" I asked.

"You're herniated!" I'd never heard her sound so alarmed. "The colostomy is prolapsed."

"What does that mean?" I asked.

"It means that it's hanging out of your body, and I think it may be infected. Why didn't you tell me?"

A dread settled on my shoulders and crawled down my back. "I didn't know."

"Aren't you in pain?" She put her practiced, fearless hands on the bulky lump, then leaned back against the wall as if viewing a sculpture or painting.

"Well, yes, but I thought that was just the healing process. I thought it would all gradually shrink."

"This won't do at all." Her usually pale, perfect Irish complexion was flushed, her freckles in sharp contrast. The dread was now numbing my legs, shortening my breath. I wasn't going to ever be in control, ever be able to irrigate.

"You mean we can't do it today?"

"We can try, but it may not work. The tube won't go into anything but a nice, neat opening." I stared at her. "I hate to say this. I'm just as eager as you are. But if it doesn't happen today, believe me, everything can be fixed."

"Oh, Terry, let's not give up, please."

"Okay, let me see, how can I get your belly to flatten out. Yes, you're going to have to lie down. Gravity will help, and then maybe we can insert the tube. Otherwise there's too much tissue in the way. The stoma's just too irregular."

I lowered myself onto the tiny bathroom floor. The blue-flowered linoleum felt cold against my back, even though the sun was shining outside. I could hear, suddenly, our yearly cardinal stupidly throwing himself against the glass door in the living room.

"Jay, the bird is back," I called.

"I know." I could hear him walk toward the deck. "I've shooed him away, but he's intent upon killing himself." The morning *New York Times* thumped thickly against the glass. "Get away, you little bastard."

Bang, crash, boom. Over and over, not realizing that glass, not air, was stopping him, the cardinal kept trying to fly forward.

"Now lie still," Terry instructed. Through the top of the sleeve, she tried to gently insert the tip of the tube, almost horizontally, into the opening.

"Ouch!" The pain was awful, like putting a pin into an open wound. Only about two hundred times worse. The stoma kept shifting. It was not stable, not really connected to my belly, but moving around, the way testicles roll and alter as a man's body moves, only, alas, not nearly so pleasing.

"Sorry, but that's what I expected," Terry said, looking frustrated and worried.

Bump, crash, boom, thump. The bird was still at it. "You dumb fuck," Jay shouted. "It's a door, you idiot. Shoo. Get out of here." He was overreacting, so unusual for him that I knew he was nervous about what might be going on with the two women and the plastic gadgetry in the bathroom.

Terry and I looked at each other. She sat back on her heels as I pushed up on my elbows from the awkward, infantalizing position on the floor.

"We have to call Dr. Kelly and tell him this has prolapsed. You can't irrigate in this condition."

I put my head in my hands and started to really sob. I could see my future disappearing. My freedom. My control. I would always have this growth dangling from my body. I would always look like the Elephant Man. Trunk and all.

Jay knocked on the door. "Barbara, what's wrong? What happened? Terry, is she all right?"

"Yes, fine." She put her arms around me as I leaned against her and wept. "We'll explain in a minute." We sat down together on the edge of the tub. "It's a good thing we discovered this, Barbara. I know how you feel. We'll pursue it until it's right, I promise you."

She helped me run a prep-pad around the opening and attach a new pouch. "Do you mind if I stay alone in here for a while?" I asked.

"Not at all." She emptied the water bag and wound up the tubing. I unhooked the mesh belt and removed the long sleeve. Terry patted my head and quietly left the room.

I sat on the toilet seat cover for at least ten minutes, just bawling for a long time. Loudly. I didn't care who heard. This seemed to be the hardest part of all: longing to go forward and being halted, after waiting five months. I'd still be at the mercy of my bodily functions. I would, I supposed, always wear a pouch, but I wanted it to be for safety, not for moment-to-moment necessity.

When I finally emerged from the bathroom, Jay looked up from his paper but didn't come toward me, as if he could make it seem less serious by not touching me. "Honey, Terry has explained it. You'll get it repaired. It's just a temporary setback." He wanted to believe that. By being optimistic and trusting the doctors, he thought he could will it to be all right. Jay's philosophy: be calm, don't panic, don't push one moment into a needless crisis.

"I know, but it's a blow. What if it has to be done over completely?"

"Barbara, let's talk to Kelly," Terry said. "The solution might just be an added stitch or two around the opening."

We all had a cup of coffee and sat in silence, each with private thoughts. Eventually we began to talk of other things. Anyone want pancakes? Is cold cereal enough? Who wants the Metro section of the *Times*? Should we do a laundry this morning?

Another saga in the medical history of Barbara Barrie Harnick. An hour later the cardinal returned for a last desperate hurl at the door. A passing neighbor called, "Oh, those birds are back."

"Yes, indeed, we know," Jay answered from the window. Again, trying to be offhand, he lightly ran his hand over my hair, but I could see how disappointed he was for me. And maybe for himself. In his eyes I thought I saw the question: Is she ever going to be comfortable again? Will we ever have a normal life?

Late that afternoon we took the ferry back to the mainland. Fishing boats, praying for bluefish, dotted the autumn-blue Great South Bay. In the parking lot Terry hugged me and smiled. "I'll see you at the hospital when you come up. I'll tell Dr. Kelly that you're going to call. Don't worry about anything." Waving merrily, she drove away.

An hour later Jay and I inched along the Triborough Bridge. In the morning I'd call Dr. Kelly and start the whole process all over again. Why was this colostomy so impossible to handle? Why was the site so red and distorted? How could it be fixed so that it didn't undulate constantly around my belly?

We were listening, on a cassette, to Mozart's Piano Concerto Number 22, a piece I love intensely. It sounds, in part, like a child's music box—bright, tinkly, clear, hopeful. The soaring spirit of Mozart, the touch of Jay's hand on my knee brought me momentary calm. His straight-ahead look was strained now, just a little.

I would get through this. Wouldn't I?

CHAPTER 26

After-Play, I

A few days after the Great Irrigation Failure, the phone rang on a warm September morning in Saltaire.

"Barbara, I'm sending you a script from the Manhattan Theatre Club." It was my agent, Scott Landis. "It's called *After-Play.*"

"Who wrote it?"

"Anne Meara."

I sat down at the picnic table on the deck. "Annie's written a play?"

"She has, it's superb, and the role for you is a dream."

"We're old friends, Anne and I. We were in Uta Hagen's acting class about a hundred years ago. And our kids grew up together on the West Side."

"I know. She'd really like you to do this."

"You've read it?" I asked.

"Yes, and I saw a workshop reading a few months ago at the Manhattan Theatre Club."

"How was it?" I walked toward the steps to shoo away a large deer that was about to eat my basil plant. "Get out of here, you dork," I yelled. The stolid buck just stood and looked at me without moving. He thought he was a pet, that I'd feed him, as many people, illegally, infuriatingly, do.

"Barbara, what's going on?"

"Oh, Scott, forgive me. It's our usual daily deer invasion. They're all over the place. Please go on."

"Are you okay?" he asked.

"Yes, really. I'm used to living with deer. Just angry about it. They'll walk into the outdoor shower with you if you let them. Tell me, please, about the play."

"It's amazing. It's about a reunion of two couples."

"Yes? Who am I?"

"Renee. She's the wife of a forced-out comedy writer. She's caustic and funny, has a horrible relationship with her kids."

"Oh, Scott," I said, still gesticulating with no effect at the deer. "You know I'm no good with one-liners. And I never think of myself as sophisticated. Renee sounds sophisticated. Is she?"

"She is, and so are you."

"This sounds like a huge stretch for me."

A slightly exasperated sigh from Scott. "It's a bit of a stretch, Barbara, but not that much. That's the beauty of it. You'll have to work hard, but you've never played a part like this before."

"Is this a firm offer?"

"Definitely. Rehearsals in mid-December, opening on January 31."

"What about the other play downtown? You know, I had lunch with the director last week, and I really liked her."

"Oh, Jean Connor, yeah, but I told you not to commit to anything for another few days."

"I didn't. I just expressed interest, but it's a provocative play."

"I knew this offer was coming," he said, "but I couldn't tell you."

"Scott! You kept me in the dark? I had lunch with Jean while you were waiting for another offer? God, I feel terrible, I just wasted her time."

"No, you didn't. You might have done that play. There was no other way to do it. The MTC had sworn me to secrecy. Besides, you were the one who would have to make the final decision. Read Anne's play now, and then we'll talk. I'm sending it by overnight mail."

After-Play was hilarious, with a subtext of heart-wrenching sadness. There was one line, about an elderly couple in a fatal automobile accident, that was so funny it made me double over in my deck chair and laugh to the trees and the birds—there was no one else around.

That weekend Jay read the play. I could hear him laughing, too, at almost the same place. I opened the screen door.

"'She was behind the wheel, and he was crossing the street'?" I asked.

"Exactly," he said, wiping his eyes. "It's outrageous."

Then he read the other play I was considering, which was very long and took him most of the next day. Over dinner we discussed both projects. And in bed that night, after making somewhat preoccupied love:

"Honey, I don't think you have a real choice," he said, tucking the light blanket around my shoulders. "Anne's play is unique and well constructed. Your role isn't like any you've ever played before."

"That's Scott's argument too. It'd be a challenge. Oh God, I'm so thirsty."

"I'll get some water," said Jay. "Look how nicely I treat you."

"How do I play those first moments when everything that comes out of her mouth is so negative?" I called into the kitchen.

"You'll find a way," said Jay. Ice tumbled into a glass. "And don't forget, it's a work in progress. There'll be a lot of changes made."

"Thank you," I said, as he handed me the water. "I guess I really should pay for this good advice."

"Oh, yeah?" He smiled. "When?"

"How about right now?"

"Honey, I'm an old man!"

"I've got cancer, and you're protesting?" He limped, like an exaggerated Quasimodo, to his side of the bed.

And we stayed up a little longer.

*   *   *

Eating breakfast on the narrow front porch: "But what do I say to the other theater?"

"You tell the truth. You thank them for the offer and say that you found something you like better."

"Oh, Jay, I hate to hurt Jean Connor's feelings."

"Barbara, it's cruel, harsh show biz. Try to be a grown-up."

"Okay."

Biking home from the tennis court: "That other play is fascinating, but it's just too long, Barbara. There's no focus, the center keeps wavering."

"The director told me that the author would cut, that she'd be at all the rehearsals," I said as we rounded the corner of our street.

Jay waved to a neighbor, "Hi, Pat."

"Hi, Jay. You guys have a good game?"

"We did," he answered. "Thanks."

We put the bikes back in the rack. "Honey," Jay asked, "didn't you hear that she's never been able to rewrite or cut any of her other productions?"

"Yes," I said, sighing.

"So you'll do that play and come home each night fuming and frustrated. I know you. You'll be on the phone for hours with the director, begging for changes. You'll be absolutely right, but nothing will happen. You'll cry and get angry and lose your appetite. Then you'll wail, 'Why did I ever agree to do this?' Don't do that to yourself. Besides, you'll be just miserable to live with."

Folding the laundry: "I think I may be able to impart my little 'message-to-the-world' with that role," I said as I shook out a pair of damp socks.

"I'm certain of it. You should do the play," said Jay. "Whose polo shirt is this?"

"Aaron's," I said, taking it from him. "He must have forgotten to pack it."

Aaron and Jane had just returned to Los Angeles after a week's visit at the beach. "Jay, did I tell you what Aaron said to me when we walked him to the ferry?"

"No, wasn't I there?"

"You and Jane were ahead of us on the boardwalk."

"Barbara, why are you redoing the shirt?"

"Because you do such a sloppy job. Why, in thirty years, can't I get you to press down as you fold? The heat of your hands takes the wrinkles out."

"Said the bishop to the nun," he replied. "Tell me what Aaron said."

"I asked him how he felt now that I was more or less out of danger."

"That's a loaded question. What did he say?"

"He said he was determined to feel okay. What do you think that means, Jay?"

"I think it means he's going to get on with his life now," he answered. "We have to do the same, so hand me that stack of pillowcases, and I'll put all this stuff away."

Explaining my difficult decision, I wrote a grateful letter to Jean Conner the following week. And on a rainy, freezing day in December I took the subway to the Manhattan Theatre Club production building, about as far west on 16th Street as you can go before falling into the Hudson River, and started rehearsals for *After-Play*.

CHAPTER 27

Back to the Drawing Board

"Yes, it is herniated, isn't it?" said Dr. Kelly, as he looked one more time at the colostomy. Terry and I had made an appointment to see him as soon as it became apparent that the operation had gone wrong.

"I think so, Dr. Kelly," she said.

He lightly pushed against the skin around the stoma. "Hmm . . . well, I guess we should do something about that."

"Such as what?" I asked, propping myself up on my elbows.

"Well," he said, "there are two ways to go. We could do an entire new operation, or we could just restitch around the opening, reinforce it, as it were."

Oh, no, not another complete procedure, I just couldn't bear it.

"Barbara, how do you feel about that?" asked Terry, immediately noticing my distress.

"Would the reinforcement work, Dr. Kelly?" I asked. I made up my mind that I would not cry, no matter what he said.

"Probably," he said, "but of course there's no guarantee about any of it. Sometimes a hernia will present itself again, sometimes not. If you want to avoid a new operation, it's the best thing to do."

My throat caught, my eyes stung. I looked down at the dangling thing flopping over my abdomen. "You do agree, don't you, that this is not right, that it shouldn't look like this?"

He smiled. Impossible to believe, but he smiled. "Well, yes, it is hanging out there, isn't it?"

I wish he had expressed greater enthusiasm about the hernia repair. I knew the only thing to do was to deal with logistics, so I said, "When can we do this?"

"How about next week?"

"Terry, will you be available, or are you lecturing somewhere?" I asked.

She took my hand, communicating instantly her understanding of the situation—that I needed her for support. "No, I'll be right here," she answered.

"Talk to my secretary, and she'll schedule it," Dr. Kelly said over his shoulder as the door closed behind him.

We made arrangements for the operation and a one- or two-night stay at Columbia Presbyterian Hospital for the Columbus Day weekend, October 1994.

CHAPTER 28

The Hernia Repair

OCTOBER 8, 1994

Columbus Day weekend was warm, the air was the bronze-gold of a Rembrandt landscape. A few red leaves, like secrets, were hidden here and there among the still-green trees. The water, reflecting the perfect sky, was periwinkle blue, and the sailboats lilted lazily, their passengers in shorts or bathing suits and white caps.

I am not describing Saltaire, Fire Island, but the view from my window at Columbia Presbyterian Hospital. Heartsick, lonely, missing the solace of my comforting community, my extended family, I was recovering from the hernia repair that Dr. Kelly had completed on Friday. He had stitched around the colostomy as if it were a piece of loose patchwork that needed to be placed back into the quilt.

I had insisted that Jay leave for Fire Island after the operation. He'd return on Sunday. After all, this was just a little interruption, a small procedure. Why should he sit by my bedside when he could be outdoors in the sun? He was preparing tours of a dozen different productions, and he'd been working long hours. He had objected, worried that I'd be lonely, but I knew from the weariness in his face that he needed a rest.

People always warn you never to go into a hospital on a weekend. A holiday weekend is even worse, deadly. The staff is shorthanded, the services are almost nonexistent, the food is a swill-like afterthought. But this operation needed to be done. The pain and the inconvenience had become unbearable.

So here I was with a roommate, lately on drugs, who wouldn't let me open the window and slept beside it for ten hours a day. Long and skinny, like a Modigliani painting, Angela had staggered into the emergency room with a uterine infection that, combined with a previous identical infection, had now probably rendered her sterile. The few hours she was up were spent frantically cleaning everything: her bureau, her bed, her pocketbook, her night-table drawer, her shoes, her fingernails and toenails, her body, her hair, her feet, the floor in her part of the room.

"You had this same thing before?" I asked.

"Sure, I knew what it was right away." Scrubbing vigorously with wet paper towels, she was lying flat on her stomach under the bed.

"How do you get it?" I squatted down to look at her.

"God knows, honey, I live on the street. So does my man. Anything can happen." She handed me the paper towels. "Would you squeeze these out in the bucket for me?"

Was she kidding? I didn't want to become involved in a cleaning fest. I started to prepare my indignant statement. And then I squeezed out the paper towels.

"Are your parents in New York?" I asked as I handed back the soggy gray mass and rose slowly, my hospital gown getting caught on one heel, so that I almost fell over. "Ow!" I said, clutching the footboard.

"You all right?" Her head appeared from beneath the bed.

"Yes, thanks." My heart was shuffling off to Buffalo. Good God, what if I had fallen with this newly stitched colostomy?

"My parents kicked me out a long time ago. The first time I stayed in this hospital, a nurse had to give me a token to leave. My mother wouldn't come and get me."

"What do you mean, she 'wouldn't come and get you'?"

"Just what I'm saying. She said she was through with me because I never behaved right." She shimmied into view now, stood up, and grabbed the bucket.

"How old are you, Angela?"

"Nineteen." With all her cleaning equipment she was on her way to the bathroom, her gigantic silver earrings swinging jauntily.

"Did you finish school?"

"Are you kidding, honey? I got to the fifth grade."

"What will you do now?" The toilet was flushing, there were sounds of more scrubbing.

"I don't know," she called out. "Probably look for a job. I got to get me a job." She returned to the room and began to dust the dresser top.

"Angela, would you consider opening the window for just a little while?" The Lysol fumes in the closed room were beginning to sting my nostrils and eyes, and it was becoming painful to breathe.

"Oh, no, honey, the air out there is rotten. I don't stay in no room with an open window."

In defeat, I retreated to the solarium.

When the fabled boyfriend arrived, she drew the curtain around her bed, and they lay there together for hours, eating potato chips, candy, Cheez Whiz, cake, and cookies. The smell of pot was unmistakable, and when he finally left, she emerged glassy-eyed, bent over and conked out on what was clearly more than just marijuana.

Recovery from the operation seemed easy. After all it had been just a repair. The rounds were made by a holiday-reduced team of interns and residents; after a first visit Friday afternoon, Dr. Kelly didn't seem to be around. On Saturday, as the covers were pulled back and the young doctors leaned over my body, I said, "When can I go home?"

"Oh, not for a while, Miss Barrie. You have a persistent fever of 101, and we can't let you go until we find the source."

"Okay, are we going to do tests or what? I seem to have a very nasty discharge."

"What kind of discharge?" asked one of them.

"A vaginal discharge." What did he think?

"Oh, uh . . . well . . ." This was clearly not in the bailiwick of young surgeons-to-be. There was quite a lot of shuffling, clearing of throats.

"This is probably a result of the radiation," I said, "but shouldn't we find out if that's the cause of the fever? Or do some more blood tests? Could it be a staph infection?"

"We have to check with Dr. Kelly, and we don't know when he'll be here."

That was Saturday afternoon. But Dr. Kelly did not come into my room that day or Sunday morning. No release, they kept saying, until the fever diminished.

My ache to be outdoors was physical. My bones and my skin mourned for the waves, for the soft air in Fire Island. I might have been cooking dinner with Jay now, the October sun flooding the village with valiant, late-season light.

A friend called, and by now I was in frustrated tears. "Tell them you want to see the head surgeon—whoever it may be—who's on duty now," she said. "Tell them you are not going to be ignored. You have to be your own advocate and make a fuss."

"But there's actually no one in authority around this weekend," I said as another boat sailed by.

"Just ask for the head surgeon. Trust me. I've been in enough hospitals. You'll get action. I'll call you back in an hour or so."

I summoned the one nurse on duty and demanded to see the surgeon in command. My voice was loud, I was trembling. No one was paying any attention to me. My roommate was now attacking the mirrors with Windex, and I wanted to go home.

In less than an hour Dr. Kelly was in the doorway.

"What is it you want?" he asked me.

"I want tests done so that we can find the source of this fever so that I can leave here."

"Why did you call the head surgeon?"

"Because you haven't been here since Friday afternoon, and no progress is being made. My bed hasn't been changed in over a day, the bathroom is filthy, trays are left here overnight, and my roommate [who was showering again] gets drugs delivered to her here and won't stop cleaning the room. I'm going crazy."

"I'll get your room changed," he said, "but what is it you want first?"

"I want to see a gynecologist, and shouldn't we do a sonogram or take some kind of picture of this procedure you've just done? I can't lie here for another two or three days and be told I'm running 101 while drugs are being delivered to this poor girl who won't let me open a window."

"All right," he said, standing up abruptly. "We'll take you to see Dr. MacMillan downstairs—he's head of gynecology and obstetrics—and we'll do a sonogram. And I'll talk to the desk about changing your room." And he was gone, without a good-bye, without a word of sympathy.

My friend had been right. The "squeaky wheel" proverb certainly seemed to be working here.

Terry Haus arrived. "You're in the hospital today?" I asked, utterly, immediately more calm.

"Yes, I had an emergency. I had a feeling I should come and check on you." Always psychic, sensitive Terry.

Two hours later, Terry at my side, I was wheeled into Dr. MacMillan's office a few floors below. He was in his late seventies, cold as a winter afternoon as he took my history. Terry filled him in on both surgeries. She was like my mother taking me for my first diaphragm.

After the examination and the swabs, he said in an edgy voice, "Well, I've never seen anything like this."

In some forty years of practice he had never seen a discharge like mine? "Could it be causing the fever?" Terry asked.

"Oh, I just don't know. It's a mystery to me. I'll give you a prescription for sulfa. Fill it out when you go home. I don't think it will do much good, but you can try." He answered his phone then and left us standing awkwardly in the room. The appointment was over.

I never filled the prescription. Terry and I went back upstairs. "I wonder if he's been told I'm a difficult patient," I said. "Was he punishing me for something?" Terry didn't reply.

The sonogram was done late that day. "It all looks okay to me," said the technician. "The exterior is a little swollen and red, but that's to be expected."

That night, as a brilliant harvest moon rose over the Hudson, Angela's boyfriend visited again. They giggled and smoked and ate for hours behind the drawn curtain. Smoke filtered through the closed-windowed room, and candy wrappers littered the floor. I complained to a nurse, but no one came to stop them.

I took my book to the solarium and waited for him to leave. At midnight I returned. Angela was asleep and stayed that way until Monday afternoon, a bucket of dirty water and a mop propped against her chair.

Monday morning the surgical resident appeared in my room. "Well, you still have a fever, so we want you to stay," he announced. "The sonogram appeared normal, but we have to find the source of the temperature."

"I'm not staying," I said. "I'm putting on my clothes, and my husband is coming to drive me home. And you're letting me out of here, or I'm going to start screaming until your ears fall off. Take your choice."

He signed the release, and Jay, fuming and concerned, walked me out of the hospital. "You do what doctors tell you," he said. "You trust them, you believe in them; and then when they desert you, there is just total disenchantment."

As I left, Angela was polishing her shoes, the ghost of marijuana fumes clinging to the blankets. My fever was never explained and disappeared in a day. The glowing, fall, Columbus Day weekend was gone forever.

A week later I was wildly uncomfortable, the stitches pulling. Back to the hospital. "It takes time," Dr. Kelly said, peering at the repair. "I'll see you in a few days."

Three days went by. The pain was awful. Back again to Dr. Kelly. "That's kind of odd," he said, " Warm water might help."

In late November 1994 the hernia repair had become a logo for a science fiction horror film. Once more I returned to the hospital, and Terry joined me in the examining room. After an interminable wait she went to find Dr. Kelly and in about five minutes returned with him.

"Oh, yeah, there's a little irritation there," he said. "I'll give you a prescription for it." Could a prescription possibly heal this swollen, ragged, obscene thing?

"Why is it still protruding like this?" I asked. "It's got to be hanging almost two inches down. It looks like a penis!"

"Oh, a little edema," he said. "Everything will eventually retract." Terry, I noticed, was not speaking, just gazing at us with an inscrutable expression.

"I'm going to Canada in a few weeks to do a television show," I said. "Can you give me the name of someone in Toronto in case I get into trouble?"

"Well, let's see . . . can I have my secretary phone you . . . or send . . . oh, well . . ." (a big sigh) ". . . wait a minute. I'll be right back." He left the room.

Twenty minutes later he returned and thrust a piece of paper into my hand. "This guy is good. He's at the University of Toronto. Call him if you want. But you'll be fine. Good-bye. Good luck."

Terry walked me downstairs. "I wonder if he's dismissing me, Terry?" I said, putting my hand over the bulge in my skirt. I wanted to be sure the adhesive was tight around the opening. I was still not irrigating; anything could happen.

Without speaking, she kissed me good-bye, and I started toward the subway.

CHAPTER 29

An Episode
for Television

TORONTO

This year the snow, surprising even the Canadians, had been early and heavy in Toronto. The air was headachy cold, stinging my face and fingers and toes into submission. The snowdrifts blocking my frozen trailer door had to be shoveled away by the second A.D. (the second assistant director) each time they needed me on the set.

I was playing a woman of sixty—an attractive woman who falls in love with a man her own age. It was a rare piece of writing: Women over fifty are usually conceived as being so old that they have no looks, no sexual desire, no vitality, no original, intellectual, or humorous thoughts, with bent bodies that lack muscle tone or strength. I felt that if I did this role properly, I'd be speaking in a small way for all women my age who have a determined hold on lives they enjoy.

During the day I had trouble walking, as each step was excruciating: the stitches, not dissolved completely, were irritating my skin, and the many layers of clothing I needed were pressing and rubbing against the swollen site.

Of course I didn't tell anyone, just prayed that my digestive system would behave itself and not burst through the pouch. Between each "take" I'd return to my trailer and check. I must have changed the pouch at least five or six times each day, praying that I wouldn't hold up the shooting; then I'd lie down on one of the banquettes until they called me again.

"Barbara, we need to do this scene before we 'wrap' tonight." The director was leaning over me as I dozed in my chair. I jerked awake. "I know this has been a long day, but if we finish the scene, we can move to another location tomorrow. Okay?"

Of course it was okay. I had no choice, even though it was now eight o'clock at night, and my makeup call had been at five-thirty that morning. I was touched-up and combed while the wardrobe woman smoothed and brushed my dress and patted my hem into place.

We took our places in the room. The extras were placed into position, and we started to rehearse.

It went slowly. Everyone was tired. It was late. I kept surreptitiously cupping the pouch to be sure it wasn't full. It wasn't. My costar, who shall be nameless, kept walking away to entertain the room with his so-called charm and wit, and the first assistant director, with six or seven pleas, had to retrieve him each time. Then, of course, he couldn't remember his lines and had to be prompted, which certainly stopped the flow of any emotion that might have been building between us.

Two hours later we limped through the last shot. We had all been on our feet for the entire time. The scene, I thought, lacked real emotion, real connection, which could have been revelatory between an older man and woman. It was as if two mature people had decided to live together almost platonically, in a kind of pleasant resignation. There was no moment of passion, no melding of two souls. What a pity. What an opportunity lost. But the extras, delighted by the attention of my fellow-actor, left smiling and animated.

I was not so happy "You know, we missed the 'event' of this scene," I said to the director. "This man doesn't want to invest in the surrender of these two people to each other, and wasn't that the salient point of this relationship?"

"Maybe you're right," he said as he placed his script into the pocket of his director's chair. "But what can we do? It's ten o'clock, and we've already gone way into overtime. And I'll never get him to be that vulnerable. He doesn't see it that way."

I gave up. The "second" assistant steered me, wrapped in boots, overcoat, and rain hood, back through the snow to my trailer. I undressed, checked my body and its plastic equipment, gathered all my things, and was driven back to the hotel through an opaque, blustery, blinding storm, which in Canada is appropriately called a whiteout.

Cradling the phone under my chin, I made a cup of coffee and called New York. "I think we're missing all the loveliness of the script, Jay. The director is really talented, but the actor just won't cooperate. He thinks it's a story about a macho man's holdout."

"Honey, can't you 'use' his attitude, make it work for your character? You're the best at that."

"Believe me, I've tried. I'm not his dish of tea, and he's certainly not mine. And of course I'm dealing with this stupid pain all the time. Oops, sorry, don't mean to complain."

"Barb, maybe you should ask for a longer lunch hour or at least a comfortable chair on the set, not just the usual canvas one," he said. "Don't, for God's sake, be a martyr."

"No, I really can't. They'll get scared and take less than my best work. It's too good a part," I said, "to throw away because I don't feel so tippy-top. At least I have to try to salvage what's left of it."

On the last night of the shoot, I called Dr. Kelly. "I'm having difficulty here; the repair seems not to be holding."

"What do you mean?" he asked.

"It's all puffy again and extremely irritated. Bloody, too. It moves around under my clothing." To alleviate the pressure, I had put my feet up on the coffee table, but the colostomy was bulging under the hotel robe like a small, concealed pillow. "I'd like you to take a look at it. Also, can I resume the chemotherapy? Hasn't it been enough time since the surgery?"

"I don't have to see you. I'm sure my repair is healing nicely," he said. He seemed to think everything would heal on its own. "About the chemo, you should see Mears. He'll tell you if you can start again. That's definitely not up to me."

I said, "Okay, Dr. Kelly, I'll take care of it."

Well, that was that. Now what do I do?

Hanging up the phone, I groaned to my feet. The room was chilly; the snow had turned my large picture windows into white abstract paintings. I managed to get to bed and a few days later finished shooting the episode.

Before the car came to take me to the airport, I did manage to do a little shopping. Colostomies may happen, infection may occur, blood may flow, but there is nothing like buying a new pocketbook to lift the drooping spirit. It was French, black, and discounted: I spent the per diem that had lain restless in my wallet for ten days. I also bought Jay and the children T-shirts that said "Toronto" in big primary-colored letters. I knew they would probably hate them, but I loved their bold pride and cheeriness.

And then I went home to Manhattan.

CHAPTER 30

Seeking Answers

Dr. Mears looked at the hernia repair as I sat, legs dangling, on the end of the examination table.

His face grew white and totally still, as if frozen by some cold substance. He stared at the results—swollen, ugly, oozing a puslike substance.

"I would like to have, Dr. Mears," I said, crying like a child whose mother had disappeared, "just one day without constant pain, just one day where I could get in and out of a chair without agony. Do you think I ever will?"

His nurse, Katherine Lesane, sweet-faced, gleaming with cleanliness, frowned with concern as she handed me a tissue and massaged me gently on the back.

Coming closer and bending to examine me, he said, "How long has it been like this?"

"For at least four weeks."

"It's not a happy sight, is it?" he said. So perhaps I wasn't a demented patient, a hypochondriac, a spoiled woman demanding unreasonable attention. But I couldn't stop weeping, and the nurse now handed me the entire box of tissues.

"Tell me, what should this thing look like?" I asked.

"It should be just a simple opening, more or less."

"Red, like this?"

"The little opening would be, but the surrounding area shouldn't be irritated. But of course each surgeon has his own technique."

"You know, Dr. Mears," I said, "I can't put on a pair of underpants without yelling, it hurts so much."

"I can see," he said, touching the area around the stoma.

"Ouch!" I cried and burst into fresh tears.

"Oh, Barbara, I'm so sorry. My God, it's really tender."

We looked at each other. "What do you think I should do? I really can't conceive of living my life like this."

He walked back to his stool and sat down. His maroon-striped bow tie and soft, blue shirt were the only colors in the white room. I sat there completely exposed, a novelty in our relationship, as it had always been Dr. Kelly who had dealt with the physical element of the colostomy. Dr. Mears, checking vital statistics and planning the course of treatment for the cancer, hadn't seen the actual operation for quite a while.

I felt once again like the Elephant Man—that pathetic creature—about to be thrust into some sanitarium for pariahs. Dr. Mears's kindliness and sympathy, however, allowed me to sit there exposed and chilly, although I longed to cover up my lower body and banish the stoma from sight.

Katherine and I waited. Then we waited some more. My swollen eyes were stinging; my bloated face felt like a balloon with discolored rivulets where the tears, beginning to subside now, had been rushing.

He said, slowly, carefully, "Would you like to seek a second opinion?"

Boo-hoo. That really did it. I was off again. I'd have to start over completely, tell my history to someone new, go through another operation. Katherine handed me a glass of water and smoothed my hair. "Don't cry, hon, you're going to be fixed up, you'll see," she said.

"I feel as if I don't have a doctor now," I said. "Maybe Kelly was angry that I called for the head surgeon on that Columbus Day weekend. That son-of-a-bitch, I didn't see him at the hospital for two days, they wouldn't let me go home because of a fever, they wouldn't do any tests, I had a druggie roommate, and *he* might have been angry?" I stopped speaking and looked down again at the colostomy. "You know what might have happened, Dr. Mears? He probably thought of me as an hysterical woman, and after that we just couldn't communicate with one another about anything. But Kelly said I had to get your permission to start the chemo again. I feel I'm losing time. Is this infection going to stop me?"

"No, you can resume," Dr. Mears said, jotting something on his clipboard.

"Oh, great."

He laughed out loud. "Did you ever think you'd be happy to know you'd be getting more chemotherapy?" he asked.

"Never in a million years. Everything is hopelessly relative, isn't it?"

"You can say that."

Katherine laughed too.

"You can get dressed, Barbara," said Mears. "I'll make an appointment with Dr. Jackson in this hospital. He's a terrific colorectal surgeon, and we'll see what he says. We'll solve this problem. Show up for chemo next Monday. See Karen in the office; she'll give you an exact time. Buck up, we'll find a solution."

At last I was going to get real help.

CHAPTER 31

Dr. Jackson

Terry Haus took me by the hand into the office of Dr. Jackson at Columbia Presbyterian Hospital. He was medium-tall, an extremely handsome man, with such an emotional connection that in two minutes I had relaxed and melted into his care.

As he gently pressed the area around the prolapsed colostomy, he said, "Does this hurt?"

I jumped under the slight pressure.

"That's the answer," he said. "Don't worry, it's just surface pain."

The operation now resembled a creature from E.T.'s space ship. "Should it look like this?" I asked. "Swollen and hanging down?"

"Well, it could use a little fixing," he said, staring at my abdomen.

"Would you fix it?" I asked as he kept carefully prodding. Terry walked over to the examining table and folded her arms.

"I believe I can if you want me to," he said.

"Do you see how those stitches have left that tissue all soft and twisted?" Terry asked.

He frowned. "I do," he said, "and that's why, Miss Barrie . . ." He placed a consoling hand on the sheet covering my knees. "That's why we'd have to close up that area, make a new incision and move the entire opening to the right side of the navel."

It sounded monumental, but I said, "Anything would be better than this."

"We'll do whatever we can to make it right," he said. He seemed to be a human soul just like me. "Take some time," he continued, "and if you decide you want to go ahead, we'll set up a schedule."

It was as if Moses had come down from the mountain, put his hands on my shoulders and said, "Thrust out your golden idols and listen to me."

Later that week, however, I called Terry at home.

"I think he's from heaven," I said, "and I trust him completely. But I'd like to start fresh—somewhere where I'm not going to run into Dr. Kelly in the hallway."

"I thought you were going to come to this conclusion," she said.

I walked with the portable phone into the living room. The sun was setting in a resplendent glow over Manhattan. All the furniture and pictures had become a pulsating wash, with no differentiation of wood or cloth or glass. My infinitesimal, mini-second life was floating in the world's suddenly magenta atmosphere. But it was my life, and for once since this ordeal began, I had to try to do what was best for me.

"Terry, I think I have to change venue. I've talked it over with Jay, and I don't want to be in a situation that brings any more tension for me."

"You have to do what you have to do, Barbara. I think you may be right."

"Thanks. I needed your opinion."

I wrote Dr. Jackson a note and thanked him for his very special attention and time. I explained my decision to have the surgery at a different hospital, to begin anew. I urged him not to take this as a rejection: He had been a great comfort, and I knew how skilled he was. Terry told me later that he appreciated the letter and that he understood completely. I had hoped that he would.

This felt like graduation from grammar school. I was a big girl now. I had made a decision that might have seemed severe, but I should have done it sooner. When a patient feels there is no other recourse, he or she must make the move, no matter what obstacles or negative feelings stand in the way.

One hears, "Don't leave the hospital where you have started." "Don't make waves, especially if you're a woman—people will think you're an hysteric." "Be a nice person." "How can you know what's best, you're not a specialist?"

All of this must be ignored.

A few weeks later, with my emotional tail between my legs, but knowing that I had to take action, I made an appointment at New York University Medical Center to see Dr. Eng, the original surgeon, the one I had walked away from so many months ago.

CHAPTER 32

After-Play Rehearsals

"My mother thought he was gay, but he wasn't. He was a great lover. If any person in this room repeats that . . ." I shook my finger at everyone in the rehearsal room.

"He was, yes, wonderful," said Rochelle Oliver, as she unwrapped her sandwich.

"Oh, I remember," I said. "You went with him too."

"Anyone want half of this hamburger?" asked Merwin Goldsmith.

"I dated him, Barbara," said Rochelle, "when he lived on Fourteenth Street."

"No," I said, sipping my tea, "didn't you go with him later? After 1960?"

"No, that apartment with the fireplace? I was there a lot," she said.

"So was I." I paused. "At the same time, do you think?"

Rochelle and I stared at each other. If I say our mouths were open, it'll sound like a cliché. But our mouths definitely fell open into wide, amazed circles.

"How's that tuna from the deli?" The stage manager was taking notes for the next day's luncheon order.

"It's tuna from hell," answered Anne Meara.

"You mean he was sleeping with both of you at the same time?" asked Rue McClanahan.

"He must have been. That sneak," Rochelle replied, a momentary shadow covering her face.

"How many years ago are we talking about?" asked Anne.

Rochelle and I began counting on our fingers. "Around forty," we said.

"My God," said Anne. "Wars have been fought since then. The computer was invented. And this guy is still so vivid?"

"Yes, he seems to be," Rochelle answered.

I nodded. I could see Jack's blond hair and guileless face, his sturdy body as he stood heartbreakingly still in a dance concert at the University of Texas, where we had met. "He was a remarkable person," I said.

"I'll say," said Anne, making a face.

Rochelle and I laughed and once more exchanged a glance. We had both loved, as young girls, a poetic, vibrant young man, dead or disappeared for over a decade. What might have been painful was now a shared, poignant experience. We became in that moment after all those years, real friends.

"Those days were so simple," said Larry Keith, who was playing my husband.

"Except for the terror of pregnancy," said Rue, turning from the telephone. "Remember that anxiety each month?"

Murmurs of agreement. Then a long silence. Memories hung over each fifty- or sixty-year-old head like dialogue balloons in a comic strip.

"What do you single people do now about condoms?" I asked. "Do you discuss all that stuff or what?"

"Absolutely, around the second date," said one of the assistants, opening a can of diet Coke.

"So soon?" I asked.

They all stared at me as if I were a fossil uncovered at an Ethiopian dig.

"Oh, honey, you just don't know what's out there," said Rue.

These were lunchtime conversations at *After-Play* rehearsals. We seven actors, the director, and the playwright divulged, without shame or hesitation, almost all aspects of our private lives. Some of us had never known each other before, but the nature of the play was so intimate, and the characters so revealed their deepest secrets, that the trust and lack of pretense seemed to flow into the lunch hour and coffee breaks, the subway ride home, the occasional drink or dinner after rehearsal.

Half-dozing during lunch, I was usually lying down on a battered couch during these enlightening exchanges. The every-Thursday, early-morning chemotherapy made me tired, the colostomy repair was bulging and lacerated; but no one except David Saint, the director, and Jane Greenwood, our costumer (who had to deal with the problem of covering it), knew of the illness or of the treatment. I just said I was used to napping at noontime.

About twenty minutes before we resumed work, I would fall into a deep, solid sleep, then eat my lunch at the table in the "restaurant" of the play. No one seemed to mind. They just considered me a sixty-two-year-old eccentric who could close her eyes and doze on a dime.

After-Play is about four old friends reuniting on a snowy night in a New York restaurant. They are joined by two other acquaintances, served by a mysterious waiter, and all experience an epiphany of sorts. During rehearsals David Saint let us talk on and on and laugh until we dropped into silent, side-clutching exhaustion. I wondered why he didn't stop us, but I know now that he was actually letting us discover the play and each other.

Larry Keith is the best storyteller in the United States of America. He starts with the first word of a joke, and the entire company doubles over. It's the tone of his voice, the set of his mouth, the raising of a little finger. Utterly hysterical, with the mystery of the coming punch line hanging in the air like a trembling firecracker: "Did you hear the one about the two embalmers?" . . . We were gone!

We all told jokes and dirty stories. We exchanged recipes and alerted each other to sales at nearby stores. Merwin Goldsmith helped Rue McClanahan begin a new diet. Rochelle Oliver brought me dried fruit from a store near her apartment in Greenwich Village. Lance Reddick, the youngest member of the cast, just out of drama school, let us taste some of his delicious grain salads prepared by his wife in New Haven, from which he commuted every day.

Anne Meara, the playwright, held back nothing about her family, her marriage, or her children. This play was, after all, a semi-fictional distillation of her life. She would march about, sandwich in hand, regaling us with personal, funny, shocking tales. It was as if we were sitting in on her analytic hours on the Upper West Side, her four-letter words careening off the walls like badminton birdies gone mad.

During the exploration of the scenes, a line or an actor's question would often evolve into a discussion of the treatment we all received from our parents when we'd been in grammar school or college or newly married. We'd share nightmares and dreams. And then Larry would tell another joke, or he and Merwin would burst into a tenor duet.

It was heaven.

I felt suspended in a kind of perfect essence. I was experiencing the joy of working on this exceptional piece of material. I was determined to make it a conflict-free, fulfilling rehearsal period. After all, I had almost not been there. In the last eight months I had experienced two rotten operations, leave-taking from the surgeon, radiation, chemotherapy, and the accompanying conditions: my hands would suddenly bleed from dry skin, a side effect of the chemo exacerbated by the cold weather, .

"Look at the back of your right hand, Barbara," Rochelle said one day. "You're full of blood."

"Oh, I'm so chapped," I lied. "I just need a Band-Aid, that's all." I was determined nothing would stop me from doing this play.

I had thought that *After-Play* would be an easy little comedy to toss off, but as we rehearsed, great lumps of identification and knowledge would rise up to hit me in the heart, making me cry or laugh. All the other actors were having the same reactions: This was a much more complicated play than any of us had anticipated.

I was playing a sixty-year-old sophisticated woman with a history of failure, illness, misunderstanding, rebellious children, and second love in a somewhat hostile but working marriage. It soon became apparent that from within Renee's veneer it might be possible to say something about the human condition. Isn't that, after all, why I had become an actress?

It was not, however, proving to be easy: Jeffrey Kramer had prescribed a mood-enhancer called Wellbutrin when a depression, resulting from the entire cancer struggle, had descended upon me like a truck accident. After the happiness of the summer, I had, quite to my astonishment, begun weeping on street corners, and a sense of despair dug at my throat like an animal. It's not so unusual for patients to suffer these kinds of emotional problems, although mine seemed to be acute.

I had been on the Wellbutrin for about three months, and it seemed to be working, but its effectiveness had placed me in a serene place: problems seemed less crucial, I cried less often, the sense of hopelessness was easier to bear.

In the play my character had a scene of total disclosure: Her daughter and grandchildren were alienated from her, and she had had cancer (yes, irony of ironies) resulting in a mastectomy. It was the pivotal moment for Renee. It called for a subtext of deep emotion because the more "real" an actor is, the funnier the disclosure will be. At least that's the way I have been trained, and it's the basis of my personal craft.

Mike Nichols, when he was putting Art Carney and me into *Prisoner of Second Avenue* on Broadway (we were replacing Peter Falk and Lee Grant), sat down with us one day in rehearsal at lunchtime. He had ordered his usual double-bologna sandwiches and a Coca-Cola, Art was eating his favorite chocolate candy-bar cookies, and I was downing my daily boring yogurt and snitching some of Art's cookies.

"Look, you have to play comedy as if it were Chekhov. You

have to establish the truth," he said. "If you say to the audience, 'Hey, we're really doing a little comedy here, and we all know it,' and you invite them onto the stage with you, they'll never come. You have to take the first moment of this play and do it for yourself, for what's really happening—it's a hot night, Art, and you've lost your job, and the air-conditioning is off, and you're miserable."

Art Carney, the dearest and shyest of men, started to protest. "Mike, I know myself. There aren't any words written there, but I know what the audiences want."

"No," said Mike. "You're better than that. I didn't hire the two of you because you're funny, which you are. I hired you because you're wonderful actors, and you've got to act."

Mike prevailed, and Art was as brilliant in that first silent moment, broken only by a "sigh," as he was in the rest of the play. Mike literally led me by the hand through my role. Once as I struggled to find an emotion, he said, "Put the glass down harder on the coffee table, stamp your foot, and the feeling will come." And it did.

Now, in *After-Play*, I was confronted by a complex scene in which I had to reveal Renee's misery while making the audience laugh. And it wasn't happening.

David Saint pulled me aside one day. "Sit down with me a minute, Barbara." We put two rickety chairs together in the corner of the freezing room. I draped my fake fur "prop" coat over our knees.

"What's up?" I asked, although I knew what he was going to say.

"Is there anything I can do to help you get where . . ."

"Where I've got to go, David?"

"Well, yes," he said, somewhat abashedly. "I know how deep your emotional life on stage has always been, but . . ."

"But I'm not getting to it in that scene."

He covered my hand with his. "Kind of. I know you work slowly, but I just want to give you whatever aid you might need."

Should I tell him about the Wellbutrin? Perhaps this was the time. I looked down at the scarred, wooden floor, then back to his open face with its sympathetic, questioning eyes. No, I didn't want to burden him with that information. Not yet at least. I had a hunch that the Wellbutrin was keeping me calm, that it was blocking the triggers that had always worked for me. And the damned colostomy was stinging and burning and gyrating around as we spoke. But these were my problems, not his.

That night I called Jeff Kramer. I was frightened, I said, that I would not be able to deliver the performance that was expected of me and that I knew I could give. Should I wean myself from the drug?

"I think you need it, Barbara. This is a tough time for you, and you need to function well."

"But Jeff, I'm not functioning well if I can't act, if I can't get to my emotions. They're like muscles, they have to be used. The Wellbutrin is stopping everything."

There was a pause. There is always a pause if Jeff is going to say something I'm not going to like. "You know you complain that the drug robs you of orgasms. Are you using that as an excuse to get off it?"

"Well, I'm not going to lie. I hate having to work so hard for orgasms. It ain't no fun, you know."

"So," he said, "convince me."

"In this case it really is the acting," I said. "I'm not going to be good in this play if I can't reach into my psyche and get things going. It's exactly the same as not having an orgasm or being pregnant and never having the baby."

His silence was deafening. Then he said, "Okay, you kind of win, for the time being. We'll try reducing the drug quickly, although I'm very ambivalent about this. Your dose is so small it won't be such a wrench, but if you start to get depressed again, you must call me immediately. Even the play's not worth your sinking down again."

"Yes, it is," I said. "I can 'use' the depression."

"Oh, you actors," he answered. "It's amazing what you'll do."

"It is," I said. "It's important. I can't fake emotion. I can't pretend that something is happening when it's really not."

"But how do you know what the emotion is?" he asked.

"That's it, I don't know, I have to find it. It sounds corny, like every interview of every actor you've ever read, but I have to experience it in rehearsal to learn what it feels like."

So with Jeffrey's halfhearted blessing, I stopped the Wellbutrin almost immediately. There didn't seem to be any side effects. I began to feel the emotions of my pivotal scene seeping through and under and between the lines—very gradually, as if I were coming to life after being asleep a long time.

Renee and I, becoming one person at last, were struggling to confess while at the same time trying to maintain a dignity. And I felt sure the laughs would eventually come directly from the character's behavior.

It felt ravishing. It was, as any actor will tell you, just like having an orgasm. Eli Wallach once said to me, "You know, when I'm supposed to be sad on stage, and it works, I'm just thrilled. To be crying makes me so happy."

As the drug left my body, the rest of my "score" for Renee began to shape itself too. David Saint was very relieved to see that I had broken through the emotional barrier. Jeff Kramer monitored my progress, and I just kept working.

This winter of 1994–95 seemed to be a perfect time. There's no doubt that I was in terrible pain, some of it so awful that I've blocked it out. (I only remembered it recently when I reread my journals.) But the elimination of the Wellbutrin, I believed, had freed me, and the cancer had somehow hollowed out my acting technique—taken away all the "junk." If I had to find a "subtext" for a moment of behavior—that is, the meaning beneath the words—it just happened, not the first week, not the second, but with time it just fell into place, as in Renee's big confessional.

Other problems were interesting too. For example: We were struggling with a scene where my husband begins to disclose his own demons. Larry Keith, sexy and moving, was close to finding this "beat," but I had a kinesthetic, subliminal knowledge that something, for me, was not right.

At one point David Saint had asked me to get up and comfort Larry, but my lines were really exposition—that is, they further explained his misery without propelling the story forward: I couldn't find a subtext for the necessary words, and I felt useless. (It's called "egg on the face." I felt covered with it.)

For weeks I rose from my chair, went to Larry, and promptly forgot my lines. Over and over, day after day. My beloved colleagues groaned and rolled their eyes each time I "went up," the theatrical term for the hellish moment of not recalling the words. I knew that if I couldn't remember anything, something might be wrong with the writing, but I couldn't convince anyone to explore that possibility.

"No, Barbara, you just have to try to drill it into your head," said David, and then Larry would tell an uproarious story about a sixty-year-old woman who couldn't remember where she had put her postmenopausal baby. And we would all howl for ten minutes, take a coffee break, and tell more tales of forgetfulness.

Finally, having moved from the hall downtown, we were about to open at the Manhattan Theatre Club at City Center on 55th Street. It was a cold, snowy day in January, and wrapped in coats and scarves, we were slogging through an always-endless technical rehearsal, which is not essentially for the actors but for the technicians and stagehands.

"Here comes the place where I have to get up," my brain registered in alarm. I tried to do it. I actually got to my feet, then sat back down and burst into wrenching, unstoppable tears.

"It just doesn't work," I cried. "You have to trust me. If I keep 'going up' in the same place, something is wrong. I can't do it. Please help me." I felt so selfish, as if I were swallowing the air around me, taking it away from the other actors.

Everyone rushed up. Our young stage managers, knowing me well, ran to get coffee and tissues. Larry gave me his handkerchief. Merwin Goldsmith put his arm around me. Rue McClanahan's eyes grew wide with wonder.

Anne Meara came onto the stage, her red hair flying. "Why didn't you say something before? I can fix it. It's easy."

"I'm so sorry. I don't mean to make a scene, but I've been complaining for weeks," I moaned. "My speeches are too perfunctory. The scene is too direct. People don't speak so sensibly in such situations. Can't we break up the dialogue so that it's more fragmented, unfinished?"

"Of course we can," said Anne, waving her arms and striding back to her script.

And that's what we did. David guided us through new blocking, Anne slightly changed the order in which we all spoke. I could now remember the lines, and I can say somewhat proudly that the scene as a whole was infinitely better. Everyone agreed.

I think the illness had wiped out the obstacles that stand in the way of work. Stripped down, exposed, my body and my soul had perhaps joined in a no-nonsense strength that made things clearer, simpler. Why fool around when the truth pushed against me like a fist and made me know that something was not organic? Why waste time when I didn't know how much time I had left in this world?

Five years ago I would have suffered, complained, and made everyone miserable. But now the path seemed unencumbered. My sensibilities were honed. And I was becoming emotionally close to a group of fellow artists who were enriching my life.

The cancer had done that. I was very grateful to it.

CHAPTER 33

Dr. Eng Revisited

On January 27, 1995, I went back to see Dr. Eng. The pain had become too intense, and the colostomy too unmanageable.

I felt stupid and humiliated, like a refugee from a cult group, imprisoned and brainwashed for months. Dr. Kelly may have believed I would be just fine, but I was in distress.

Once again I was out in the world.

Even as I reached up to hang my jacket on a hook in the waiting room, the misshapen colostomy, covered awkwardly by my skirt, brushed up against the wall like a scraped, worn tennis ball. Trying to stop the burn, I quickly clutched myself and, hiding my face, counted to ten until the stinging subsided.

It was a good thing I had come here today—things were getting worse.

Dr. Eng, small and neat, was reserved and slightly judgmental as I brought him up to date. This was not my imagination. As I sat in his office and told my tale, he asked few questions, his fingers moving over his lips, sometimes averting his gaze.

In the examining room Mrs. Kucynski joined us, and she, too, was noncommittal, her face innocent of any emotion. What did it take for her to be sympathetic? Were these two people going to forgive me for being so foolish more than six months ago?

"Charlotte [so that was her first name], can you help us pull up this gown?" asked Dr. Eng. From the other side of the table she peered at the stoma, and I saw her express what seemed to be total shock.

She moved closer as Dr. Eng just looked down. He didn't touch me, he didn't say anything, he didn't move. He just stared. Charlotte's eyes were riveted to the colostomy. She was waiting for Dr. Eng to speak.

Walking toward the foot of the table, he began to press the area around the stoma. Still he said nothing. Then he sighed. Charlotte's body softened into a less militant posture. I suddenly realized that she was a beautiful woman, slim, with highly defined facial bones, no makeup, a long neck, eloquent hands. The barrier between patient and nurse began to evaporate.

Her empathy was like a suddenly radiating warmth. What I had perceived as coldness, I now understood had been clarity: She had dealt with hundreds of patients and had to keep her objectivity until the problems had been delineated. Now I felt that I had a supporter, someone who might help me through this crisis.

I waited. More prodding and gentle manipulation, but each time Dr. Eng touched me I inadvertently let out a half-strangled bark. More sighs from Dr. Eng. More frowns and understanding glances from Charlotte.

When I could no longer bear the suspense, I said, "Dr. Eng, do you think you can fix this?"

He kept his head down. Charlotte stood still. The room began to close in, like shutters, as if the next remark he made might actually blot out the light and keep me forever paralyzed in this condition.

"Well," he said quietly, after an interminable silence, "it has to be better than this."

We all sighed in unison. The truth was out: Something had to be done. "Get dressed, Miss Barrie," he said, "and we'll talk in my office."

"When do you think you might operate, Dr. Eng?" I asked as I sat down near his desk.

"We should do it as soon as possible, but I hear you're in a play."

"I am," I answered. "Can we wait until the closing? It's March 5."

"Can you deal with the discomfort?" he asked.

"I can," I said, "but will I be in any danger? I mean will the whole thing fall out of my body or get damaged?"

"No," he answered, smiling. "Just keep it supported with a light girdle or something like that. And of course you can't irrigate until it's fixed."

"I know," I said ruefully. "I've tried, and it's just impossible."

"Yes, it would be," he said, his mouth turning down in slight disdain. "But you know, you must learn to do it later. It's the only way for you to really live well, and I'm going to insist on it."

I leaned forward. "Dr. Eng, please believe me, I've been waiting to irrigate."

"You'll find it will change your life," he said, as Charlotte came into the room with her clipboard. He rose and walked around to my chair. "Make all the arrangements, and we'll do our best, I promise you."

Charlotte, warm and concerned, discussed the operation date, which would be March 7, and told me what to expect: the preexams, the approximate length of stay (about ten days), the insurance forms. Dr. Eng's wife and children beamed from their framed pictures under the window, the East River boats beyond churning narrow trails of white water. A helicopter rose from the 23rd Street landing pad and made its way toward Kennedy Airport or a destination farther out on Long Island, maybe even my beloved Fire Island—all this visible movement as I sat in the black leather chair, planning yet another period of immobility and enclosure.

But surely this time it would work.

CHAPTER 34

Before the Third
Operation

FEBRUARY 27, 1995
ALMOST TEN MONTHS FROM THE FIRST OPERATION

I was on the treadmill again. New thallium stress test for the third operation. If my heart was strong and the arteries unblocked, we would try to repair the really bad colostomy. (The angioplasty had been a year and a half earlier: I was probably a compendium of ills for the record books.)

After-Play was about to close, and there was strong talk about reopening at a new, larger theater. This was the perfect time to enter the hospital.

After being injected with a dye and walking on the treadmill at NYU Medical Center, I would be on my own for two or three hours. No food, no liquid. Just water and Jell-O or clear broth. I was already starving, as no nourishment is allowed twelve hours before the test.

When I returned to the hospital, I was to lie under a machine that would photograph the heart and surrounding area—the "thallium" part of the test. From the dye, a picture, rather like a watercolor, emerges, and the heart is evaluated: Has the stress revealed a blockage or other irregularity?

In a few days Dr. Eng would be operating to redo the entire colostomy. He would be moving it from the left side of my body to the right side. New location. Fresh, untouched tissue. Elimination of the hernia. Smaller bowel opening. No more pain. We hoped.

Once more, strange hands had lifted my breasts to paste on the holders for the wires that would record all my statistics as I walked on the machine. It didn't seem to matter. I was so used to being totally exposed a lot of the time. But what if these breasts, too, became infected? What if the cancer had already deposited a tiny cell there, so tiny that even a CAT scan couldn't find it? I couldn't imagine living with a mastectomy in addition to a colostomy. Wasn't there some kind of alliterative joke there? Or "How much could a human bein' stand?"—a quote from some book or play about country folk? Or that phrase, "God doesn't give us more than we can bear"?

Oh, yeah?

More needles in my arms for various reasons. More pasted stickers to record blood pressure, heartbeat, and so on. I wanted terribly to pass this test so that I could be approved for the operation. The hernia had grown to giant proportions, and the stoma was often bleeding and looked more prolapsed than usual, if such a thing could be possible. In other words, the bowel was now hanging out of my body more than three inches. It emanated from a round aperture about four inches in diameter. Yes, it looked exactly like a pink penis coming out of a doughnut. Really charming.

In an effort to hold in the whole thing, I now wore only latex panties, but they seemed not to be effective; and by evening I was usually in violent pain, as the area around the stoma was stretched and bleeding from changing pouches throughout the day.

However, I had sailed through *After-Play,* and never during this wonderful successful production did I feel any pain while on stage. How could that be? To put on the black stretch tights each night I had to lie down, covered with a blanket, and pull them up as I gazed at the ceiling. I was resisting gravity, of course: It was the only way to push down the hernia and the bowel and keep them there. It was an awkward procedure, complicated by trying to keep it secret from dressing-room mates. I had told them that it was a garden-variety hernia, but Rochelle Oliver told me later that she intuited exactly what had been going on but had decided to give me my privacy.

Once the play began I forgot it completely. The wine-colored suit, sensitively designed by Jane Greenwood, had an overblouse and a jacket that moved freely and concealed the telltale lump. When I changed back into my street clothes, I could find out in the bathroom how much the pouch had filled. (Oddly enough it was never very much, as if my body knew that I was busy doing something else.)

By bedtime it had done its job and had to be changed again. The entire area had to be cleaned, prepared with the special little saturated pad, and when it was all dry, the new pouch attached.

This was generally accompanied by tears and curses, covered by music from WQXR turned up to an obscene volume so that Jay couldn't hear me.

Some of the abominable attacks I have forgotten, but when Jane and Aaron were visiting in January 1995, I evidently did one of my screaming-fainting acts after the show one night.

"It was one of the times I got really scared," confessed Jane in the summer of 1996, on Fire Island. "Don't you remember, Mom, you came in the door and kind of went down to the floor on your knees?"

"No, I can't . . . oh, yes," I said, "and Daddy and you led me to the sofa in the library . . ."

"And we brought you a vodka, neat, and you cried and cried, and finally after you drank it all, you fell asleep."

"Yes, it wasn't too happy a time, was it? You must have been very upset," I said as we rounded up our books and hats and towels for a trip to the beach.

"I was for a while. I knew the operation was bothering you, but you were doing the play, and you did seem to be recovering, but . . ."

"But you have to admit," I said, "that it was really the pits." She nodded. She had clearly been disturbed, but it was only now, over a year later, that she mentioned it.

"Jane," I asked as we left the deck, "do you think you and Aaron have had effects from the cancer stuff that we've never discussed? I mean, do you think because I was in denial that you've held things back too?"

"All of the above," she answered. We stopped to pick some blueberries from our bushes along the walk.

"I'm thinking again about that first phone call," I said.

She popped some berries into her mouth. "Oh, the one that you and Daddy were not going to make?"

"Don't rub it in, honey, but yes, that one." She picked some more berries for me. They were slightly tart and very hot from the sun. "I've always wondered how Aaron could have been so brave. I knew you were crying, but I've never seen him wilt, not the entire time."

"He did, he did," she answered, "we both did, but after that first call, after he put down the phone, I started to say, 'What are we going to do? We should go back, she could die,' and he had already started to become emotional, and he tried to hide it. And he said, 'Hold it, hold it,' and he went into the bathroom."

"How long did he stay?"

"Just a few minutes," she answered as we descended the wooden stairs over the dunes, "but we stopped working, I think. I just went home."

We settled into our rusting canvas chairs and gazed together at the slowly rolling breakers. To our left, perhaps an eighth of a mile away, was the Broadway Beach, where most Saltaire parents take their children to play in the surf under the watchful eyes of the lifeguards.

But here on our West Walk Beach, the "No-Talking Beach,"

as my friend Carole Sirovich calls it, I was sitting next to my daughter, silently. We watched a cloud become outlined in gold as it slowly drifted across the sun. It was a blessing that I was here today in this exquisite place. But would I ever understand what my family had gone through? Did I need to understand it? There may be parts of the story that will never be told. Maybe that's best.

Another evening during the run of *After-Play*, some of the actors went for a drink to a quiet restaurant on Seventh Avenue, near the theater. Suddenly while we were talking, twelve sharp knives seemed to fly into the hernia. I stopped speaking or hearing, doubled over, and started to cry.

Larry Keith put his arm around me and bent his head close to mine so that no one else could hear. "Barbara, what is it . . . what *is* it?" he whispered. From the emphasis on "is," I knew he had probably been aware for a while that something was amiss.

"Nothing," I lied. "I have a little hernia that acts up sometimes."

"This reaction doesn't seem so little."

"Yes, really, I just need an Advil or two."

Bob, the waiter, hurried over. "Miss Barrie, are you okay?"

"Of course," I said as I struggled to regain my vision. Who was I kidding? Everyone at the table looked concerned. "But do you have an Advil or an aspirin around?"

"No, but I'll get it for you," and in a moment he was out the front door of the restaurant.

Hoping that no one could see how bad this was, I kept my head down and changed the subject. Don't ask me what we talked about . . . the performance that night, the audience, a dropped line, a woman in red in the front row whose beeper kept zinging. But I deflected attention for a few moments until Bob came trotting back with the bottle of Advil.

He pulled out the cotton and placed two pills in my hand. "This should help," he said, carefully not looking at my face, which now featured two puffy turtlelike eyes. I felt like an infant, an idiot, a spoiled brat, a 128-pound weakling.

By the time I walked into our apartment an hour or so later, I fell into Jay's arms and really screamed. He led me to our bed, where I lay on my back and bawled loudly for a very long time. I no longer cared if the neighbors heard me. I only wanted the twelve knives to be pulled out. Jay brought me water, and I sat up against his arm and drank what I could. Finally after taking another tablet, the pain subsided somewhat.

"It started in the bar," I said.

"Why didn't you leave right away?"

"Because I want to be a perfect person, that's why."

"You don't have to be so brave, Barbara," he said.

"I know, but I just don't want people treating me like a cancer patient. Isn't it amazing that these attacks never happen on stage?"

"Thank God for the play," he said. "It's your therapy."

What had carried me along? Why had I been so fulfilled in this role? So thrilled to go to work every day of rehearsal and every night of playing? During the run of the play Jay and I had discussed it many times.

One night late in February we were in our bedroom. Having become a "Court TV" addict, I was watching the O. J. Simpson criminal trial. Jay was engrossed in a new script.

"Jay, I am going to have a severe postpartum depression when this play closes on Sunday."

"And when this damned trial is over," he said.

"You're right," I admitted.

"But then you'll get repaired, and you're going to be Hercules's mother. [I had just been hired by Disney as a "voice" for their next animated film, Hercules.] And I've reserved a tennis court for us the Friday after the operation."

"Oh, goodie, I'll be there. But may I talk to you for just a moment about this cancer thing? Oh God, Rosa Lopez just made a joke about her friend and the kitchen. This woman is unbelievable."

"Barb, it's me or O. J.," he said, putting down the script. "Take your pick."

"Okay, okay . . . wait now." I sat up straight and pointed to the screen. "Look at her face. Are those lawyers paying for her grandkids' education for the next hundred years or what?"

"Barbara." He just hated this new obsession of mine, the trials, the discussions, the late-night phone dissections with other crazed viewer friends.

"Sorry." I turned back to him. "Here's what I want to say. Would you think I'm insane if I say that this illness has given me many gifts?"

"Not at all. I can see it in your behavior. Cancer patients say that often, don't they?"

"Yes, and I used to scoff at it. How could such a thing be true? But now I think I've distilled the whole experience into an image."

"Tell me."

"I feel as if my body is outlined by a big, soft, black crayon, but the outline is about six inches away from me. Like a Keith Haring drawing, you know? And there are openings here and there in the outline, and the air in my soul whooshes out to meet other people's real selves. Not their facades but their true souls. I can see them so clearly. And weather. I embrace the weather every day. Cold or raining or snowing . . . I love walking in it. Oh look." I had heard something startling. "Christopher Darden just made Rosa say she could have seen the white Bronco around nine instead of eleven. He just wrecked her alibi. Where was I?"

"Barbara," said Jay, "I'm losing my mind."

"But honey, she contradicts herself in every other sentence. You've just got to watch this."

"Please finish this conversation," Jay said. "Forgive me, but I'm really tired and I've got to read this script."

"Yes. Well, I listen better than I used to. I react more viscerally, especially since I'm off all the tranquilizers, and that's tough sometimes. I mean, I'm crying at card tricks again—so overwrought about everything all the time."

"But darling," he said, "that's the way we know and love you."

"You never take me seriously, Jay. Don't you understand? I appreciate people more. I think I'm much kinder. I do treasure my life, but you know I've never been bored for a moment—oh, maybe the two days before Jane was born—I was so fat . . . oh, watch . . . Johnnie Cochran is going to do a redirect."

"Barbara, you have one more minute." He clamped down his hand on my shoulder. "I love you, but my eyes are closing."

"But do you get it?"

"I do. You are something totally out of this world. I don't know how you've done it. The operations, the pain, the chemo. And you're brilliant in the play."

"Really?" The actor's ego . . . forever active.

"Yes, really. Now kiss me good night because I have a tennis game in the morning, and, as you know, nothing is more important than that."

"Would you like a really important kiss, or do you actually want to go to sleep?" I snuggled up and lifted the worn cotton of his pajama top.

"Honey, you are the dream of my life, but the fuck is definitely off."

"Okay. I'm going to watch O. J."

I had passed my stress test with ease. Everything was normal. My heart doctor was jubilant. Dr. Eng was relieved. I was told I had the physical capacity of a fifteen-year-old girl. (So why do they keep telling me I'm sixty-three?) And that night, two days before I entered the hospital for the third time, Jay and I took a steamy shower (my children are going to hate reading this), drank red wine, talked lazily, and made love.

As usual we had to be careful of my painful left side, where a blessedly clean pouch was making plastic noises.

And I kept saying, "Don't look. Don't look." And Jay said, "It's actually very cute, that bag. It has real style. Let me see."

"*No!*" I tried to cover that area, but I was giggling.

"Barbara, it doesn't matter at all. It's become the part of you I love best."

"Thanks a lot."

"You're welcome."

Later, much later, during the time we would have smoked a cigarette but no one does that anymore, I said, "What if I only have a year left? I won't get a clear bill of health until next May at least."

"Honey, you're going to be like your mother. You'll live to be ninety-seven." His hug was full of conviction. "Let's pray, however, that you don't turn out the way she has."

"Do you think there's a danger in that?"

"Of course. But with nineteen years of analysis you've so far managed to avert it. Well, most of the time anyway. But the possibility is there, ever waiting."

"What would you do if that ever happened?"

He yawned. "Leave you in a nanosecond."

He waved a hand in my direction as he turned over on his side, but he was already half-asleep. "Good night, little honey."

I read for a while. *Patrimony*, by Philip Roth. It's about his relationship with his father. An exquisite, almost perfect book, like a Picasso line drawing, so uncluttered and direct.

The end, when I reached it, was devastating. Philip Roth had lost his cherished father. I had lost mine, but at a much younger age. Still, when a father dies . . .

We all suffer these crises and losses, burst into sweat when the phone rings too late at night, pray that no harm befalls those we love. But it does sometimes. Philip Roth's father grew very, very sick. Like me.

I had lost part of my body. And I had a lot ahead of me, and it wasn't going to be fun, and I might be taken away from this husband and these children forever. Then again, I might get lucky and, as Dr. Mears had said, "beat this disease."

I turned out the light and lay in the dark. In two days I would enter the hospital for the third time. But tomorrow I would report for the closing performance at the Manhattan Theatre Club at seven-thirty P.M., the usual half-hour. I'd do the play, give my little "message to the world," maybe go out with friends afterward, laugh, tell stories, walk home along Central Park West, make grocery lists, brush my teeth, listen to Vivaldi, all that stuff.

Astounding. Just astounding.

CHAPTER 35

After the Third Try

MARCH 1995
NEW YORK UNIVERSITY HOSPITAL

Dr. Eng's interns clustered around him every day at my bed-side. Often they would come from surgery, some still in their blue, wrinkled gowns, their eyes blurry from endless days of work with too little sleep.

Not Dr. Eng. Always cheery, smiling. "How are you feel-ing?" he'd ask, his blue turbanlike hat tilted forward.

"Great," I'd say.

"Me too. I'm great. I did a great operation here," he beamed, looking down at my belly. "Look, you see," he said, drawing back the sheet, "just a rosebud. That's the way it should look."

The medical students peered groggily at the new colostomy. It was true. There were steel staples on the left, where he had unwound my bowel like a garden hose and sewn up the herniated muscles and skin. He had pulled the intestine under the skin to the other side of my navel. There he'd made a tiny opening, about as big as a dime, so that it looked as if I had two belly buttons, both "innies." It was a revelation, a miracle, not to have that huge, repulsive appendage protruding from my body.

There were three incisions now: the old stoma and hernia repair, the original middle incision from the first operations, and the new stoma opening. I looked as if a tic-tac-toe board were imprinted upon my body. It was somewhat sore and not a lot of fun. Only this time I didn't have to have my rectum removed. It was already done. So I was one step ahead, if one could look at it that way. I never thought I'd ever say, "Thank God, my tush is already sewn up." How one's perspective changes.

"When can I have some food, Dr. Eng? I'm fainting from hunger."

"Oh, very soon. But I want you up, up," he said. Behind him a pleasure yacht was anchored at the water's edge, and the busy lines of traffic on the East River Drive wove like lines of ants in either direction. My window looked like a drawing from one of Richard Scarry's transportation books for kids. "You must walk around and around the halls. If I come in again and find you in bed, I won't let you go home for a long, long time."

The young people were glassy-eyed now, longing for breakfast and a bed. One girl gripped the footboard as she trembled with a yawn. "Okay, I promise, I promise," I said.

The next day I was given water, Jell-O, and ice pops. "Why am I so fortunate?" I asked the nurse.

"Because really what you're eating is just water. We feel pretty safe about that."

The beauty of small things: the moisture, the taste of the cherry Jell-O, the coolness of the popsicles against my lips and throat, water with ice, the springtime flowers that arrived from friends. Gradually I was put on real food, a complimentary term for the rubbish that was delivered on my trays. But my strength increased, and I was beginning to walk with some pace around the corridors.

The blue-coated gang, exhausted as usual, arrived late one morning. Dr. Eng, chipper, energetic, happy, had already operated twice since dawn. "Miss Barrie, have you started irrigating yet?"

"No, not yet. You know, I couldn't do it before because of the other operation."

"But now you have no excuses. You must do it right away. You're like any other person in the world," he said, grinning. "You can do anything that anyone else can do. But this procedure will free you. One of the nurses will teach you how."

A young, half-Irish, half-Chinese, utterly beautiful nurse hustled me into the bathroom two days later. She filled up the water bag and hung it on a hook over my head. She helped me fasten the plastic sleeve around my waist with a stretch mesh belt. She tried to teach me to insert the tube into the stoma, but it was like torture, and I felt nauseated.

"I think I may throw up," I said. The gray tiles were dancing in a hula line, up and down and twirling around.

"That's usual, Miss Barrie. It gets to be a routine after a while." And we had a long conversation about her dog and how it was taken care of by her parents, who didn't want to tell her when it finally died.

"Can you imagine that I didn't even go to the burial?" she asked. "And he was my dog for years before I gave him to my parents. Isn't it awful that they didn't let me know he was sick and then that he passed away?"

"Awful," I said, as she flushed the toilet and wiped the seat with a wet paper towel.

Trying to be brave about this and feeling utterly naked and disgusting, I attempted to make conversation. No dice. I leaned over with sharp cramps.

"Does it always feel like this?" I asked.

"The cramps? Oh, sure," she answered, holding my shoulder, "but you'll get used to it. It's a good thing actually. It means the water is going in."

She left me alone for a while with the plastic paraphernalia extending around and above me like a Rube Goldberg contraption. This was a low point. It was smelly and excruciating, and I felt, really for the first time, crippled and wounded.

How could I ever master this? And then go out and rehearse a play or do the marketing or go to the Philharmonic? Or, God forbid, make love or go swimming? I would be chained to the bathroom for how long? How many hours a day? What if it never worked successfully and I had more accidents like the one that day on the Broadway bus?

When the nurse returned, she looked at what must have been my anguished face and said, "Now don't get discouraged." She unhooked me from my plastic entrapment. "You're going to conquer it. You'll see."

Maybe. But I was going to call Terry Haus as soon as I got home.

Three days later I was given a release from the hospital.

I was going home, on my way out of a nightmarish year. In spite of it all I had had my second book published; and I had done a successful play, which we were going to reopen in May; a Movie of the Week in Toronto with Meredith Baxter; another Movie of the Week in Vancouver (with Tony Randall and Jack Klugman); a television episode in Toronto; two After-School Specials for ABC Television; and *Scarlett*, the mini-series for CBS Television.

I had played tennis and had a summer on the beach, cooked some interesting (and not so interesting) meals, spent time with the kids, entertained friends, been entertained by them, cursed and yelled at my wretched operations, laughed a lot by the fireplaces in Fire Island, made love (once under the stars in our outdoor shower, glasses of champagne resting on the little bench).

If I could do all that in the midst of three operations, three hospital stays, and radiation and chemotherapy in between, surely there was hope that I could finally become a repaired, useful person.

If I could just learn to do the goddamned irrigation.

On subsequent visits to Dr. Eng's office, Charlotte emerged as another angel in my life. I was required almost every four or five days to report there, where she answered my questions with the utmost understanding and caring, her aquiline face responding with sympathy every time a new problem arose.

"How is the irrigation coming?" Dr. Eng asked during each visit.

"Well, it's getting better," I said, although I knew that the ultimate management of the water bag and the nozzle and the plastic sleeve was still not complete.

"Yes, you keep at it. You're going to be a liberated person if you do."

He had entered the room on crutches, the result of a late-season ski accident. "Dr. Eng, you're not so free yourself."

"Oh, listen, they wanted to put me to bed. I said, No way. This will heal. I've got patients to attend. Can you imagine me laid up?"

No, I couldn't. "Dr. Eng, can we talk about my sexual life?"

Without skipping a beat, he enthusiastically replied, "Oh, *yes*, absolutely."

"Am I allowed to resume? I mean I'm not talking about swinging from chandeliers or anything."

"By all means you can swing from chandeliers," he said, and we both laughed. "Just wait a week or two and swing away."

Until he felt certain that I was healing and that the irrigation had become doable, Dr. Eng kept me coming back for visits. His attention to detail was compelling. His manner, unostentatious and direct, gave me confidence that I was going to be able to live my life.

"You know," he said, "I didn't trust that initial central incision you had gotten, I just didn't trust it, so you see I never touched it. I went underneath and pulled the bowel through. I don't want you to think this area around your navel is weak. It isn't. You can be sure the area is stronger than ever."

Charlotte, standing by the supply table, nodded. She knew how good a surgeon he was. And then, "Okay, Miss Barrie," he said, "see you next time, keep up the irrigation. I'm going to pursue you until you get it right."

CHAPTER 36

Irrigation

APRIL 4, 1995
HOME FROM THIRD OPERATION FOR 3 ½ WEEKS

It's not irrigation of the fields or gardens. It's irrigation of yourself—an enema every day—through the new opening, or stoma (the word that I really hate), of the bowel on your belly or near your hip. Wherever the doctor placed it.

I know. It seems unthinkable. It is, for a long, long time. Some people elect never to irrigate—perhaps because it is time consuming or a bit technical, or for various other reasons. Deciding to let nature take its course, they empty or discard the pouch when necessary. This is perfectly acceptable. It is just a matter of choice.

This is how it works: You take a long, graduated plastic tube that looks like an overextended dress sleeve. Two inches from the top is a plastic ring that you position over the stoma. The sleeve is secured by an elastic belt that hooks into small openings on each side of the ring and goes around the waist.

You fill a calibrated hot water bag with warm water and hang it above, but not too far above, your head—usually on a wire hanger or two, through the double-reinforced hole punched into the plastic. From the bottom of the bag extends a long, narrow tube. At the end of the tube is a perforated (with one tiny hole) plastic cone that inserts neatly into the stoma.

One hopes.

Seated on the toilet, with the sleeve hanging into the bowl, you release the water (anywhere from 500 to 1,000 cc's) by placing the cone through the open top of the sleeve and into the stoma. When that's completed, you fasten the top of the sleeve, just like a Ziploc bag.

Then you wait while your intestines begin to give back the water mixed with stool. (Hang in there, reader, it's just facts, not as bad as they sound.) You flush the toilet often and clean the sleeve by pouring water through it from any capacious bottle or pitcher, which is refilled when necessary. In a while you can put a broad plastic clip at the bottom of the sleeve, tuck the whole thing into the belt, and walk around the house while making beds, doing laundry, or writing a book. It sounds a bit strange and smelly, and I'm afraid it is. But you can get a lot of chores done, and in forty-five minutes to an hour it's all over.

After that the sleeve and the belt are vigorously washed in dishwashing liquid and left to dry over a towel rack. The water bag is flushed out and the cone cleaned. Then it's time to wipe up the bathroom with Lysol, take a long shower, and wait another twenty-four hours to do it all again. Some people irrigate once every other day and wear only a little plastic pouch or a Band-Aid.

Ha. (I'll see about that!)

At first this was such an unimaginably difficult thing to do that it made me furious. A strange object is inserted into a place in my body that was never meant to be invaded. A contraption that reduced my spirit and made me feel like a coal mine: the sleeve was the chute through which matter was being expelled.

Because the first two operations had both herniated, it had been physically impossible to insert the cone, and the attempts were excruciating. From the failed experiment on Fire Island the preceding September, I had had to wear a pouch and trust to luck for almost a year.

In late April of 1995, I was hesitant even to begin. I loathed the thought of fooling around with my body and its products. Let the pouches take care of it—I would go my merry way.

But then one night after Dr. Eng's operation had healed, my angelic friend and nurse, Terry Haus, came to the apartment to attempt once again to teach me the steps. It seemed insurmountable: The water wouldn't go in immediately, then it did and nothing happened. We sat in the bathroom and waited for results.

"Terry, how can you bear to do this? To muck around with other people's excretions?"

"It's just shit, Barbara," she said, smiling. "We all have to do it for ourselves anyway." She settled back into the small chair we had brought into the bathroom.

"But still, doesn't it become tedious and unpleasant to be around it all the time?"

"Not when I see all the good I can do. I visit people, especially old people who are shut into their houses, who think there's no hope for them. Anything happening there with you?"

"I feel gurgling and a little cramping."

"Oh, good. Good." She leaned over and adjusted the plastic sleeve so that the circle covered the opening more evenly. "We're on the way."

"Oh, great. I know I'm going to be thrilled."

"You will be when you can do this once a day and forget about it."

"You're right. I'm sorry."

"Don't apologize. Everyone feels this way the first time." She moved to the mirror above the sink. "Boy, do I need a haircut. What do you think? Don't I need a haircut?"

"Oh, Terry! Something's going on here." The premier gush of the first irrigation in almost a year. It may sound fairly alarming, but I was very pleased. I couldn't believe that something was finally happening the way I had been told it would.

She put her hands on her hips and gave a rolling Irish laugh.

"See, I told you."

"This is what it's like?" I steeled myself against the clutching at my side, like a hand twisting my intestines.

"Yes," she yelled. "Hurray for you. Now we'll sit and chat and wait for the second stage."

"There's more?"

"Oh, sure." She filled an empty seltzer bottle with water and handed to me. "Now we'll open the top of the sleeve and pour this down."

"I wondered how I cleaned this thing," I said.

"Well, there's no need to sit there with all that stuff. Just keep filling the bottle—here, you can lean right over here to the faucet—and pour it down until the sleeve is nice and clear."

"You're a phenomenon, Terry. I can't thank you enough for all this."

"Barbara, it's my job," she said as she sat back down on the chair.

We settled down to wait for the next . . . whatever. I didn't know what to expect.

"How do you feel?" she asked.

"A little woozy, but okay." There were tears pressing against the back of my eyes. "It's so unsettling, this experience."

"Yes, you got it. It is."

I leaned back against the toilet lid. This was the oddest scene: the nurse and the patient, both waiting for a new bowel movement. And talking, primping, and laughing. They don't make up stuff like this!

"These people, Terry, the ones you help, what do you do?"

"Oh, I have to scrounge around. First I find someone who will pay for the supplies—insurance companies, welfare agencies. Some of these people are so poor they can't afford to buy anything."

"But how can anyone survive without the pouches and the belts and all? I mean, how can they go out on the street?"

"Barbara, you can't believe what people can do. They use rags and stuff their underwear and never go out. They live isolated, frightened lives."

"Oh God."

"But I can teach them how to take care of themselves. Anything else coming there?"

"Maybe in a minute," I answered.

"Good. Let me see." She poked the plastic sleeve. "Yes, this is going to be just right."

"Gee, thanks."

"Or someone will come from South America who's never seen a doctor. We arrange an operation and instruct them the way I'm instructing you."

"Who pays for that?"

"Various agencies. Often the hospital." She pointed at my belly. "Oops. Now it's flowing. Wonderful."

Another cramp buckled me over. Not so bad this time, and the results were gratifying. Terry kept right on talking. "We had a patient from Ecuador who had had the operation, but it had gone wrong, and he was spewing feces all over the room. He'd been doing that for months."

"Oh, Terry, do I want to hear this?"

"Sure you do." She turned on the faucet. "Let me fill the bottle again."

"Thanks."

"Here's a story for you: A kid came from Russia who'd been run over twice by a bus in the Urals. His leg was broken so badly that it had atrophied in a bent position. His urinary tract was smashed, and he needed an ileostomy, for the urine, you know . . ."

She handed me the bottle but remained standing, animated with enthusiasm. "The notion of making a new body opening for urine was beyond the doctors in Moscow. They told the mother, Sasha, to bring him here. She wrote letters and sold everything she owned. Her rotten husband washed his hands of the whole thing, so she literally carried the boy in her arms from Moscow because by that time he couldn't walk at all. We found an agency that would pay for the operations—there were five of them, all done at Columbia Presbyterian."

"Where did they live?"

"With me. Where else?"

"You had them in your small apartment?"

"Why not? Isn't that the way we're all supposed to treat one another? We had an amazing time."

"Terry, you're really something."

"Nonsense. They're remarkable people. They live in New Jersey now. Oh, hear that gurgle? That means you're almost through." She actually clapped her hands. "He goes to school, Peter, the kid, I mean. He's just brilliant, and the mother is working. Only in America."

We cleaned the sink and the toilet with Lysol disinfectant and hung the sleeve to dry. Over an hour had gone by.

In the living room Jay poured me a stiff, neat vodka, and Terry had a little glass of wine. We all sat around the dining room table and ate the Chinese food delivered from the local restaurant: vegetable dumplings, spicy chicken, sesame noodles, and sautéed green beans. Here I was, eating. And tomorrow I would have to do this whole procedure over again. Was I crazy? Wouldn't it be better to fast or starve?

Can you believe this tale? Can you believe that colostomy patients can learn to do this and go right on, with their souls intact? Irrigation must be incorporated into one's life. What time of day should it be done? What if there's a little leakage afterward? (There usually is at first, until one gets used to the feel of an empty intestine.)

What about traveling? Well, you have to use bottled water in certain countries, and since the luggage often gets lost or delayed, you must carry extra equipment with you at all times. And check it, in panic, about fifty times before the plane lands. And drive your husband crazy. Bad enough to constantly lose spectacles and subway tokens and airline tickets, which always slip between the seats. But life-allowing pouches? The consequences are too devastating to imagine.

As the green April days passed and *After-Play* was once again in rehearsal, I knew I had to get the routine down. Gradually I did. I learned to take the portable phone into the bathroom with my reading materials and old towels to throw on the floor in case of accidents.

I could watch the O. J. Simpson trial from the set on my desk in the bedroom. I could answer the phone and read *The New York Times* or paint my toenails. While waiting for further evacuation, with the clip on the bottom of the sleeve, I could walk around the house, make beds, vacuum, work at the computer.

Something began to change: My body began to function in its own new way. Even the much-reduced fragrance made me feel that I was alive, not dead as many of my relatives were, although God knows I would have preferred to defecate in the old-fashioned way.

Now I can go out for the rest of the day and the evening with a pouch on as protection. No accidents (well, rarely), no embarrassments, no odor, no bulge beneath my sweater. I'm able to walk onto the stage and wear leotards and one-piece bathing suits, and no one can tell that underneath is a flat, dun-colored pouch. Dr. Eng doesn't think I need to wear one at all, but I tell him, "Just convince me of that, with hundreds of people staring at me from the audience."

After all, any of these operations could have left me permanently damaged. I can see, I can hear, I can work, play tennis, swim, make love, run. I can work on this book. I have the joy of Jay and Jane and Aaron. I'm what I always wanted to be: a wife and mother, a working actress, and in the last five years . . . a writer.

That's not to say that my life is like the *Ladies Home Journal* articles. Hardly. I have disappointments, Jay and I argue about a lot of things, I have blue days and sometimes troubled nights, we worry about bills like most other people, and we have to adjust to the effects of aging, which are continually startling and unbelievable. (Who is that white-haired lady staring at me from the shop window. Oh, good heavens, it's me!)

Nothing will ever be the same. Nothing is the same now. I will always have to take at least an hour each day and deal with all the appliances and the waiting and the cleaning and the wondering if I have been successful this time. Did I securely press the adhesive to my belly so that if I should have an occasional emergency, the pouch will hold?

I am freed from the former tyranny of my illness. And, need I say, the tyranny of death. I have to keep my perspective, right?

CHAPTER 37

After-Play,
Second Production

On May 2, 1995, one year to the day of my first bungled operation, we reopened *After-Play* in a different theater—this one
on 55th Street called Theater Four. The cast was the same
except for Rue McClanahan, who had had previous engage-
ments. Anne Meara was now playing her role.

We were again a huge hit with sold-out houses on weekends and solid ticket sales during the steamy weeks of the
record-hot summer.

When rehearsals had first begun, there was a discussion
about what time we should gather each morning. Start
early and leave at four? Or avoid the crowded subways and
arrive at ten o'clock?

"Well, I have chemotherapy every Thursday at ten, so I'd
appreciate being called as late as you can on that day," I
announced.

David Saint stared at me. Wasn't I keeping this secret any
longer? No, I was not. The third operation had given me a
new passport for living, and I was just accepting the chemo
as another activity in my busy days.

The two new stage managers nodded their heads, although
they were clearly stunned by the revelation. She has cancer?
Is she going to be able to do this? Is she strong enough?

Trying to remain cool, they said, "I'm sure we can work

that out" and then started outdoing themselves in reaching for pencils and papers, chattering, they thought, nonchalantly, but making quite a lot of noise.

Cancer scares people. They are frightened for themselves and for you. I suppose I should have taken them aside earlier and delivered the facts, but I have to admit it didn't occur to me: I was by this time so used to living with my condition.

Every Thursday morning for nine months I had ridden the subway up to the oncology room at Columbia Presbyterian, where diminutive, lively Allison Kimberg-Kern would take my blood for testing. After the white blood cell count was approved, she administered the chemotherapy solution from a bag placed on an IV stand above my head, a process that took about twenty-five minutes. If I was in a hurry, she'd give me a "push," just inject the solution right from a syringe directly into my arm.

Allison often sat with me and we'd talk about the latest philharmonic concerts, the theater, the exhibits at the Metropolitan Museum of Art. She and her husband lived across the river, in Rockland County, and were culture inhalers, coming into the city for as many events as they could.

Over the period of a year's treatment, she became another person who helped pull me through. Often, when we began to run out of veins to stick in the needles for the blood samples or for the solution, I would crumple into tears: My skin would scream, but more importantly, my spirit was beginning to shatter.

"Barbara, I understand," Allison would say, putting her trim arms around me. "Just sit here, and we'll be quiet for a moment."

Meanwhile the other supersensitive nurses in the room would scurry around to bring me orange juice, tissues, water, a pillow for my back. "Barbara, it's all right," Susan Vogel, another nurse, insisted, her wise brown eyes gazing into mine. Everyone patted my shoulders and wiped my forehead. "This is normal, don't worry, everyone goes through these times." Energetic and positive, they were like the other halves of their patients: the sturdy, wise, healthy, alternate parts of these sick people, about whom they so visibly cared.

It's such a draining job to treat—to deal with individuals who indeed will get better, but also dealing with others who may die much sooner.

Every day. Hundreds of blood tests and needles and IV bags and tears and pain. They were always smiling, without fail—clearly knowing that what they were doing was important and healing and would make a palpable difference in the world.

Each Thursday as I walked into that room, I saw glowing halos above their white-uniformed, sweatered bodies. When I left I always had the courage to face my day (and in this case, the night, where I was performing on a stage!) and to return the following week.

During that summer run of *After-Play*, I learned that the day *following* the chemotherapy was the day I felt weak and nauseated. And if I was taking the additional pills—the Ergamisol—on the second day at exactly four o'clock in the afternoon, I would double over, the sidewalk or the buildings or the kitchen walls heaving and crashing down around me.

Jay asked me to meet him at a 57th Street gallery one Tuesday. He wanted to see some black and white drawings by Willem de Kooning, an exhibit that would soon close. "Lovely," I said. "Will you treat me to lunch too?"

"I wouldn't miss one thrill-packed moment," he replied.

After lunch we went up in the elevator to a quiet, empty, small gallery. As we walked around the two rooms, I began to feel the Ergamisol Nightmare begin. Perspiration formed behind my ears, my arms started to shake, my breath was hard to catch, and worst of all, I felt that I was going to vomit.

"Jay," I whispered, clutching his seersucker sleeve, "can you find me a chair? I'm passing out."

He had been through this before. "Oh God, it must be four o'clock. Is this your Ergamisol week?"

"It is," I said as I sank into a molded plastic chair that the receptionist had quickly provided.

"Put your head down, honey," he said as he knelt down and held my legs.

The first sensation produces weeping. Just weeping. It's uncontrollable and seems to be a symptom, not a result, of the temporary sickness. One feels so helpless and so full of despair. Would I ever get well? Would I ever get off these killing drugs? Would I ever stop collapsing in public places?

The waves of nausea gradually diminished. The carpet beneath me was spotted with my perspiration and tears. "Anything else I can do?" inquired the frightened receptionist, who thought, no doubt, that she was going to have a dead, bloody body in her black and white gallery.

"No, thank you," I said. "It's going away. I'm so sorry."

"Please, please, don't apologize," she assured me. "I just feel terrible that I can't help."

Forty-five minutes later I was feeling, as usual on these occasions, much improved. Jay bought me a Coke with lots of ice, which was the antidote of choice. We parted with a kiss, and I went on to Theater Four where I lay down in the dressing room and slept until "half-hour," the time when actors must check in and begin to get ready for the performance.

Greg Fletcher, our stage manager for the second production, told me just recently that on the day after the chemo or on the second day of the pills, the staff knew I would be affected. Through a little window on stage right they would watch me with concern. Was I going to make it? How ill did I seem to be this week? Was it the week with or without the pills? If it was a matinee, how would I do at four o'clock when the poison kicked in? ("Poison" was exactly the word Dr. Mears used when he finally took me off the Ergamisol in the fall.) "You've had enough," he said. "Your body won't take any more. It's a tough medicine. It used to be for deworming sheep, you know."

"Now you tell me?" I gasped.

"I wanted to go easy because some people don't have severe side effects."

"But I . . . ?"

"You did," he said, "but the worst is over."

Now I said, "Greg, I never knew you watched me. How kind of you all to be so attentive."

"Well, that first day of rehearsal, when you announced your chemo schedule, we were worried about you," he said. He had come to our apartment to help me straighten out my computer, which was always getting too cluttered with my inefficient methods. "We didn't know how you got through it, Barbara."

"Oh yes, it was pretty scary, I guess."

"Do you remember that you used to come offstage with your 'usual flair' and then hit your head against the brick wall and start to slide down?"

"Come on, Greg! I did?"

"Yes," he said as he rearranged something on my computer screen. "Gosh, you can really louse this thing up. How do you manage to make such a mess?"

"Because I'm a Jewish person," I replied, "and I don't understand machines."

"I'll say. Anyway, we'd bring you water and sit you down, and then you'd recover quickly. But it was so hard for us to see you suffer like that."

"It was all of you and the work itself that got me through," I said. "Is it too late to thank you now?"

His cherubic face looked up from the keyboard. "You can thank me by paying more attention to your Headers and Footers. I put them in for you, but you're not using them."

"I hate my Headers and Footers," I said. "Please take them out, I'm not smart enough to remember how to do them on the new chapters."

We had all given up our summer vacations to do this play we loved, and it was a joyous run until late September when the audiences diminished, and I caught a devastating virus that settled in my vocal cords. In mid-October I left the production.

It was time for a rest.

CHAPTER 38

Lunch with Dr. Mears

"What exactly is radiation?" I asked Dr. Mears. "I always thought that I kind of knew, but I really don't."

I had never asked that question before. Now, writing this book, I realize what little information I possessed. I asked Dr. Mears if he could spare me some time.

"I'd be happy to," he said with enthusiasm. So on an early June day in 1996, we were in the doctors' dining room at Columbia Presbyterian Hospital, Dr. Mears with his welcoming, easygoing presence, and I with my yellow pad of queries.

"Radiation is energy," he said. "Electrons are the source of that energy. Cobalt was used in the early days, but it wasn't understood." He leaned forward eagerly, as if he were teaching a class. "Madame Curie stood in a box and let out all the rays, so of course all the cells in her body were damaged. Now we design a field of treatment for each individual body, the 'simulation' you had before you started treatment, remember?"

"How could I forget?" It had taken two days as intensely concentrated people in a glass booth conferred and came out to push me into one position after another.

Dr. Mears and I went to the buffet table and filled our plates with fish, pasta, and different kinds of healthful, sensible salads. As we were seriously debating, brows furrowed and chins in hands, whether the luscious avocado glistening on the plate was a good-cholesterol food or a bad-cholesterol food, I asked, "Am I seriously interrupting your day?"

"Not at all. This is great," he said, and we both took the avocado.

After we were seated again at the table, I asked, "What is the radiation supposed to do?"

"In your case, the high-energy beams are directed to the place where the tumor had been and to all the other places it might go, to sterilize the field of activity, as it were. The theory is that the DNA is damaged. Radiation treatment can eliminate worry."

"'Worry?' Doesn't that seem like a generic solution?" I asked.

"Not really." He had not started to eat: this subject, after all his years of practice, was much more intriguing to him than food. "There are concerns about reoccurrence in the pelvic area. Before radiation that was more or less the rule."

I looked up. Oh, that tumor might come back after all. I knew this, but it was shocking to hear it. I kept on writing.

"Radiation is a powerful influence. Yours was a rectal presentation, the radiation was preventive. We hope, with all radiation, that all the bad stuff is killed and the good remains."

"What do you mean 'we hope'?"

"Well, we don't know how it actually works. It's really a theory."

"A theory?" I stopped writing.

"That's right."

"But even though people get well, you're still not sure how it works?" I asked.

He finally started to eat. "That's about it," he said, almost sheepishly.

"Ah yes," I said, putting down my pen, "and some people die."

"Um, they do," he said. No apologies. It's just the way it is. I admired his candor.

"Do you mind when patients ask you questions?"

"On the contrary. It makes me nervous when a patient says, 'Okay.' I mean I've said, 'We'll do this treatment,' and the patient says, 'Okay!' But a patient who is proactive may actually help himself get better."

"You mean that stuff about participating in your own cure may not be hocus-pocus?"

"I think it's not hocus-pocus at all. Who knows? Life may be easier for the passive patient, but it's just not the right way to go."

Here I was, after all this time, asking questions, but I kept my head down as I took notes. I felt that I had been lazy and foolish. Maybe I'd thought, two years ago, that the less I knew, the less I'd have to deal with: just go along blindly and do what I'm told.

He put down his fork again. "It's a generational thing, I think. Overly aggressive young people sit there with their parents right in the room and sometimes say, 'How long does he or she have?' That's the wrong question to ask at that minute. It's important to maintain hope for those who are ill. Those insensitive people, I've come to believe, have other agendas."

We ordered coffee. "Is being a doctor all you thought it would be?"

He didn't answer immediately, but then a look of self-confidence and pleasure seemed to illuminate the air around him. "Yes, it is."

"Can you tell me why?"

"Well, you know, I did lab research for quite a long time. In 1976 the technology of the gene was just exploding. I was the first person, believe it or not, to see the DNA of a gene under the microscope."

"The first?" I said.

"I wrote papers and lectured about it—a very heady time in my life, but I missed the patients. I had become interested in leukemia when I did my residency at the Boston University Medical Center. All those sick kids, some of whom, with chemotherapy, came from the brink of death back to life. When I returned to Columbia, I kept saying to Arthur Bank, my mentor in research, 'I want leukemia.'"

"So what happened?"

"I just chose to focus on helping people get better. I gave up research and went into practice. Opened an office here in this hospital in 1982."

"Were you scared?" I asked.

"Oh, sure. I'd take anyone who'd walk in the door. But I need that interaction, the longitudinal reward of getting to know the patient." He paused. "Sometimes, as often as not, I believe I've done something good."

His beeper went off, and while he went to use the phone, I drifted back to the buffet table. There were pears poached in wine, chocolate cake, fruit salad, crème brûlée, and other temptations.

Mears joined me at the buffet. "Don't you think we should have a little dessert?" he asked.

"Definitely," I answered, "particularly since there are pears in wine."

Just then a man on the other side of the table said, "You're not going to skip the crème brûlée, are you?"

We looked at each other. I was trying so hard to be fat-free disciplined.

"Not for a minute," said Dr. Mears, and we both dived into the crème brûlée.

We ate for a while in silence. Then he gazed across the room, his eyes slightly dreamy behind his horn-rimmed glasses, and said, "You know, my mother died of breast cancer. I never thought about it until recently, but it may have informed my choices in medicine. What do you think?"

"I think it may have," I said.

CHAPTER 39

Santa Barbara

LABOR DAY WEEKEND, 1996
SANTA BARBARA, CALIFORNIA

I am playing Brooke Shields's grandmother on a new series for NBC Television called "Suddenly Susan." If I have to be a grandmother, it might as well be gracious, bright Brooke Shields's.

A week ago I had been bereft at leaving Fire Island in the middle of a perfect late-August week. I was on my way to Los Angeles to begin rehearsals for the second segment of the series. I actually wept the entire trip while the flight attendants politely looked the other way. I'm sure they thought I was having a complete breakdown.

The next morning, however, I woke in Jane's apartment with an unexpected, inexplicable decision to remain in Los Angeles and not to return for Labor Day weekend, a beloved ritual for all Fire Islanders. Had I experienced an epiphany? How had I switched so abruptly from one mode to the other?

I needed some guidance. Jane was in New York, so Jeffrey Kramer and I arranged a phone analytic hour early one morning before rehearsal.

"What's happened, Jeffrey? Why am I sure I shouldn't come home?" It was six-fifteen, and I was staggering around Jane's Santa Monica kitchen, trying to make breakfast.

"Barbara, maybe you're growing up, maybe you're beginning to understand now what hold that place has on you."

I took the bread out of the fridge and filled the coffeepot with water. "Because it's just like Corpus Christi, where I grew up?"

"I think so," he answered.

"But why am I so grief-stricken each time I leave?"

"It's only a thought," he said, sounding solid and awake, "but do you want to hear it?"

"Sure," I said as I sat down on one of the old painted chairs. Was this going to be hard to take? Sometimes Jeffrey got right to the point, but only after he had all the facts. Well, I had been seeing him for four years: He must know everything by now.

"I believe you're always looking for answers there, and now you may be changing: You know you're not going to find them."

"Oh God." Why hadn't I brewed the coffee earlier? I desperately needed it now. "You mean questions that I've had since I was a little girl?"

"Could be. You have this series. You have the book. You're realizing, maybe, that there isn't a millennium for you in any one place."

"And I'm not going to have *not* had cancer." My throat began to throb, little explosions popped behind my eyes.

"And listen, Barbara . . ."

"Jeffrey, I know what you're going to say: My father is not there, I'm not going to find him there."

"No, because your father is dead."

It was such a naked word, "dead," said without pause or embellishment. I could see it in front of me, black and white printing on a bold placard. It was unusual for Jeff to speak quite that directly, especially because he knew what an incendiary area my father's sudden death was for me. But this might be the most efficacious way—to say it out loud, no euphemisms, use the real word: DEAD.

But I knew Jeff was right. I had taken some kind of step forward. I had left, even for a moment, the deceiving comfort and fantasy of my little village and had faced the world. I had stopped thinking that my safety or my youth lay hiding in that piney, sandy place.

The feminist writer Nancy Mairs says that our lives are made up of all the houses, all the rooms, we have lived in. Our bodies, she believes, are the "bone houses" of our existences—the memories, the sexuality, the souls, the experiences we have known.

My "bone house" consisted of the apartment in Chicago where I was born, the tract house my father bought in Corpus Christi, my University of Texas dormitory room, the West End Avenue apartment where Jay and I had brought up our children, our new apartment, and the little place in Saltaire.

But I had had cancer. My father was gone, my girlhood in Texas was gone, I was married to Jay. Jane and Aaron were out in the world, and our house, while it would wait for me, was not going to restore my health nor my soul to their former states. Everything was different now.

Two weeks ago my daughter and I were dressing to go and play tennis. As she tied back her hair, she said, "You know, sometime I'd really like to see your stoma."

"You would?" I asked, surprised, looking at her through the mirror in my room. "Are you sure?"

"Yes, I'm curious."

"What if you're shocked?" I asked as I sat down to put on my socks.

"Mom, what's the big deal?"

A few days later as I emerged from the outdoor shower, I wrapped a big towel around myself and entered the house. Jane was in her room.

"Janie, want to see it now?"

"Sure," she said and came to her door.

I slowly loosened the towel and exposed Dr. Eng's "little rosebud."

She looked carefully at the spot. "That's it?"

"That's it," I said. "About the size of a dime, right?"

"It's amazing. God, Mom, what did the old one look like?"

I closed the towel. "Like a penis hanging from a dough-nut. Really, like the Elephant Man. That was the image always in my mind."

"And that's really it? That's where it all happens?" She seemed unruffled, able to take in this information without flinching.

"Yes," I answered, "but I've become very fond of this colostomy, isn't that insane? Terry Haus tells me it's because it's freeing, it's my gate to health."

"Well, it is, isn't it?" she said. "It looks, I must say, almost normal."

"Normal compared to something," I said, "but I'm not sure what."

In New York, about a month before, I had finally shown my body to Jay. "Wanna see the ole stoma?" I had asked as he was inserting a CD into the record player (I still call it a record player).

"Yep," he said. "It's show-and-tell time."

"Take a look," I said, slowly pulling up my shirt.

Jay was definitely taken aback. The little red dot in my belly felt like a beacon reflected in his eyes. His concern for me was palpable: Here is my wife, not as I first knew her, but altered.

"Are you surprised?" I asked, holding up the shirt like a banner.

"I am, somewhat, but not as much as I thought I would be. It's just that little spot, that's it?" The piano music of Oscar Peterson, one of Jay's hands-down favorites, spilled across the room.

"Yes, didn't he do an incredible job?"

"I'll say." We stood looking at each other. Then he put his hands on my breasts. "But the body, for an old lady, is still terrific."

"Thanks," I said. "Every little bit helps." I lowered the

shirt. Soft afternoon light from the city skyline silhouetted his shoulders and head. There didn't seem to be anything to say. The worst had long been over, and we were already in the new part of our lives.

Both of us, however, were still adjusting to the tyranny of daily irrigation: When to do it? Will we miss a train or a bus if I try to finish it in the morning? Is the water okay in Los Angeles, or should I use bottled? How early do I have to wake up in order to do everything and get to work in time? If it doesn't function, will I have an accident in bed at night?

Today, Labor Day, 1996, Aaron and I are ensconced in a two-bedroom guest house with its own living room and kitchen. It's a miniature Connecticut cottage, appointed so perfectly that it's like living in an America that probably never existed: toile wallpaper with pictures of boys fishing and girls on swings, couples dancing, a man driving a horse and carriage; in the rooms, simple tables and hooked rugs.

Outside, pink and purple bougainvillea climb the walls of the other houses on this estate. There are vast and varied rose gardens, mountainous California live oaks with their oddly small leaves, and English-style plantings everywhere.

Bill and Bonnie (Bartlett) Daniels are talented, beloved actors and two of our best, traveling-couple friends. These last two days we have played tennis, swum many laps in the pool, and walked up steep hills. We have watched, shouting and wincing, the U.S. Open in their comfortable den and eaten memorable meals cooked by Bill—Irish oatmeal, chicken on a spit, vegetable stew, berry cobbler, Belgian waffles, rosemary-roasted corn, and fresh strawberries.

This is a very sweet life.

I have no idea what the future will bring. The tumor may return or metastasize. I may become ill from something else entirely. Tomorrow, September 3, Aaron will drive me back to Los Angeles and then go on to Vancouver, where he will gratefully be observing John Erman direct a Hallmark Hall of Fame.

Tuesday I will "camera block and tape" the next segment of "Suddenly Susan." In a few days I'll resume my peripatetic life, flying back and forth from New York to Los Angeles until the series is complete. Soon Jane returns to work in Los Angeles, and Jay will start to oversee the many productions Theatreworks/USA has in rehearsal.

We'll have Rosh Hashanah and Yom Kippur on Fire Island, New York, or Los Angeles, depending upon everyone's schedules. The autumn colors of the sky and sea will grow heartbreakingly intense—another summer gone—more days, vivid and active, that will fade into our lives.

Jay and I, on a nippy October day, will finally close the house, defrosting the refrigerator, cleaning the oven, hiding all the candles and soaps and paper away from the mice. We'll hang our wooden wagon in the shed and store all the rusty, falling-down bicycles under a useless blue tarpaulin.

The great American poet W. S. Merwin's poem "Season" is about his home in the French countryside:

> *this blue door open to the lingering sun this stillness*
> *echoing from the rooms like an unfinished sound*
> *this fraying of voices at the edge of the village*
> *beyond the dusty gardens this breath of knowing*
> *without knowing anything this old branch from which*
> *years and faces go on falling this presence already*
> *far away this restless alien in the cherished place*

I am beginning to understand that I am a "restless alien" in my "cherished place." Always longing to find an answer, yet knowing, through this experience of cancer, that the answer is to be forever elusive. It is very frustrating, sad, hard to accept, but that's the way it is.

Yesterday I asked Aaron, "Have you forgiven me for not leveling with you about my illness, even though I did it inadvertently?" We were sitting on the little front porch of the Daniels's guest cottage.

"I have, Mom, but really, I'll never do that to my kids when I'm a parent."

"I hear you," I said.

"Yeah, but of course when I have kids, I probably won't tell them a thing."

I laughed. "Oh, Aaron, you're very special. You'll do exactly as you please."

"I suppose. But some good things did come out of all this."

"Yes, what?" I asked.

"The day of the operation, when we finally left the hospital, we went to the Dallas Bar-B-Que for dinner. I've never been so hungry, we were famished, we were in shock because it had all happened so quickly. I don't remember what we ate except that we ordered the onion loaf, just pigged out on it."

"What an understandable choice," I said.

"Well, we were a family that night, you know," he said, leaning back in the chair. "I think people's true colors come out, like in sports—the way people perform in sports is supposed to be the way they really are. It had been so frightening, but you had been so strong, *so* strong, and when we walked out of the waiting room, we knew you weren't going to die, and Jane and Dad and I really bonded for the first time in a long while." He gazed into the garden. "Did you think you might die?"

"No, I've told you, I really did not, but just in case . . ." I glanced quickly at him, "I left a list of things I love on the computer, did you see it?"

"Oh, yes," he said, turning to me. "I wondered what that all was—Yeats and Indian food and tennis."

"And Mozart, Fra Angelico, and Larry Gatlin, things like that," I added. "Now don't be upset, but I thought it would be a good idea to read it at my funeral, many years from now. Do you think I'm crazy?"

"No, no." He waved away my remark as if it were a pesky fly. "We'll do it when you're ninety-three, but Mother, listen to me." He leaned forward, almost angrily. "You could have died in New York, and Jane and I would have been in California thinking that it was 'just a minor operation.' Promise me you'll always include us from now on. We're there for you. Don't shut us out."

He put his hand briefly on the arm of my chair, and we grew quiet for a moment. The noonday sun topped the trees in a slightly hazy glow, and Bonnie's daylilies and daisies gossiped in the breeze.

We were in the middle of a William Merritt Chase painting.

Now here's the thing: I had lived to sit on an ivy-covered porch, on a resplendent California day, and have this conversation with my son.

Aren't I lucky?

Afterword

Otis W. Brawley, M.D.
National Cancer Institute

Barbara Barrie's story of courage and struggle against colorectal cancer is just one example of the challenge that thousands of Americans face each year. It is estimated that by the end of this year 131,600 persons will be diagnosed and 57,000 will die from the disease. Colorectal cancer is the second leading cause of death from cancer in the United States. Cancer of the colon or rectum strikes Americans of all races and all ethnicities. It strikes both men and women. While it is fair to say that most colorectal cancer patients are over the age of fifty, there are also teenagers and young adults with the disease.

While the number of Americans touched by this disease is staggering, major advances in the past twenty-five years have dramatically improved the chances of survival and cure. New strategies for screening and early detection show benefits in saving lives and reduce the amount of treatment needed for cure. This means today's colorectal cancer patients have a better quality of life. New surgical techniques have greatly reduced the number of colorectal cancer patients who need a permanent colostomy bag.

WHO IS AT RISK?

Everyone is at risk for colorectal cancer and risk increases with age but scientists have begun to understand and define those persons at highest risk. Studies show that colorectal cancer is much more prevalent in North America and most developed countries when compared to South American, African, and Asian countries. First-generation migrants from areas of low incidence to areas of higher incidence acquire the higher risk of the area to which they migrate. Dietary factors are thought to be the cause of

245

these differences. People with diets high in fiber and low in fat tend to have a lower risk of colorectal cancer.

About one-fourth of the persons with colorectal cancer have a family history of the disease. Persons with a family history of colorectal cancer, a history of colorectal polyps, inflammatory bowel disease, chronic ulcerative colitis or Crohn's disease, familial predisposition, and history of other cancers are at the highest risk. Persons with a history of ovarian, endometrial, or breast cancer may also be at increased risk. Some families with rare hereditary syndromes (familial adenomatous polyposis and hereditary nonpolyposis syndromes) are at very high risk for colorectal cancer.

CAN COLORECTAL CANCER BE PREVENTED?

Everyone is encouraged to eat at least five to nine servings of fruits and vegetables a day, because people with diets high in fiber and low in fat tend to have lower risk of colorectal cancer.

Studies are underway to determine if certain drugs can prevent colorectal cancer. So-called chemoprevention of cancer is a relatively new idea. There is some suggestion that compounds such as calcium carbonate or nonsteroidal anti-inflammatory drugs such as aspirin might someday be used to lower a person's risk of colorectal cancer. A number of chemopreventive agents are being studied in clinical trials.

WHAT ABOUT SCREENING?

Adults without symptoms of colorectal cancer should consider colorectal cancer screening. The most convincing studies of the benefits of screening show that people between the ages of fifty and eighty who have their stool tested every one to two years for evidence of blood (occult blood test) have less risk of colorectal cancer death than those who do not. In one well-designed trial, people who had been screened decreased their risk of colorectal cancer death by one-third. The test is painless and simple. A small stool sample is placed on a special paper and a chemical is applied to test for evidence of blood. If blood is present, the smear turns blue, and the patient may need a follow up for colorectal cancer.

Most physicians also recommend that persons over fifty receive sigmoidoscopy on a regular basis in addition to having their stool checked for occult blood. Sigmoidoscopy is an exam in which a thin tube is placed up the rectum so that the sigmoid can be examined. The exact interval for sigmoidoscopy varies; some physicians suggest the exam every three years, others every five years.

It is recommended that persons at extremely high risk or individuals with blood in their stool on the screening test should receive either a colonoscopy or a double contrast barium enema, and sometimes both. A colonoscopy is a test in which a flexible fiber optic tube is passed through the rectum and the entire colon is examined for evidence of polyps. A double contrast barium enema is a radiologic test in which a liquid barium mixture is administered to outline the colon. X rays of the abdomen are then taken. Both tests are capable of detecting small polyps or irregularities that might be considered early cancers or pre-cancerous lesions. People at high risk may choose to start screening before age fifty and may elect to do it more frequently than those at normal risk.

Medicare recently began paying for colorectal screening for persons over sixty-five. Educating the public of the potential benefits of screening so that they might seek the services is still necessary.

THE WARNING SIGNS OF COLORECTAL CANCER

Persons with symptoms that suggest the possibility of colorectal cancer should see a physician. The warning signs include visible blood in stool or dark black stool, a change in bowel habits, pencil thin stool, a loss of appetite, and weight loss. Colorectal cancer is generally painless until there is significant growth of the disease. It cannot be stressed too much that people with these symptoms should find a good physician. The first sign of a good physician is someone with whom the patient can have a conversation. Feel free to discuss concerns about colorectal cancer with your physician. Too often I have heard of patients who suspected that they had colorectal cancer for months or even years, and they saw their physicians but never discussed their concern.

THE TREATMENTS ARE AVAILABLE

Medicine has had significant improvements in the treatment of especially low-stage or localized colorectal cancer. Today, most patients treated for colorectal cancer are cured. Prognosis is far better for those diagnosed with small tumors that have not penetrated the bowel wall. Polyps and precancerous lesions that line the colon and rectum can be removed with the use or a sigmoidoscope or colonoscope. Large polyps and tumors must be removed through abdominal surgery. A pathologist examines the colon and polyps under a microscope to determine if cancer is present. The extent of surgery is determined by how advanced the cancer is. Thankfully, the surgical techniques of today allow for far easier recovery than the techniques just ten years ago. Occasionally some patients whose disease has spread in the rectum may require an ostomy. But the number of patients requiring ostomies has decreased tremendously due to the development of anal sphincter–sparing surgical techniques. This has been a significant improvement in quality of life for many colorectal cancer patients.

Patients with colon cancer that penetrates through the bowel wall and people who have evidence that cancer has spread to abdominal lymph nodes will often get chemotherapy even though it appears that all the cancer has been removed by the surgery. The use of so-called adjuvant chemotherapy became common in the late 1980s after several clinical trials showed that several combinations of chemotherapies—fluorouracil with levamisole and fluorouracil with leucovorin—prolonged a patient's survival. In addition to chemotherapy, some patients with rectal cancer may also receive up to six weeks of radiation therapy.

Colorectal cancer presents some of its greatest difficulties when it spreads from the colon or rectum to other vital organs of the body. A common site for the spread of the disease is the liver, which is all too often fatal. To date, there are no efficacious treatments for colon cancer once the disease has spread to the liver. Systemic anti-cancer treatments have been shown to prolong the time to progression of cancer but have not been shown to cure metastatic disease. Much of current research is focused on improving treatment for patients with metastatic disease—that is, cancers that have spread from one organ to another. The latest treatments being developed and tested include less toxic chemotherapies, monoclonal antibodies, and immunotherapies that train the patient's immune system to reject the cancer.

The revolutionary new scientific advances have emerged as we learn more and more about genetics and cell biology. Researchers have already discovered a number of different genes that are mutated, or changed, to cause cancer. As scientists learn more about the genes that are expressed abnormally in colon cancer, physicians will be able to better diagnose the disease and better understand how to treat the disease.

But despite the very best of treatments, many Americans are simply not benefitting from the research. Among them are special populations: the poor, the elderly, and the disenfranchised, who still do not have adequate access to screening services and, even if diagnosed, may never receive adequate treatment. We must help our relatives and friends stricken with this disease.

Much of the success in the treatment of colorectal cancer has come from the participation of thousands of people in clinical trials and studies to see if screening saves lives, if colorectal cancer can be prevented with diet or drugs, and if better treatments can be developed.

If you or a loved one need up-to-date information on state-of-the-art treatments, call the National Cancer Institute Cancer Information Service at 1-800-4-CANCER.

Sources

Once you have been diagnosed with cancer of the rectum or colon and you have sought a second or third opinion, what happens next?

The colorectal surgeon should thoroughly inform you what the operation entails and what to expect afterward. Some hospitals have ostomy nurses who visit you in your room a few days after surgery. They are terrific, a godsend, for that is the time a patient can feel most overwhelmed with all the changes that are taking place. A good doctor will always insist on many follow-up visits after the surgery, and he or she and the assistant will usually answer all the questions you may have.

In addition to your chosen doctor and staff, you may wish to call various organizations:

The American Cancer Society was enormously helpful in giving me a packet of statistics and information, facts about colorectal cancer, nutrition, exercise, etc. (Their national home office is at 1599 Clifton Road NE, Atlanta, Georgia 30329-4251. The toll-free number is 1-800-ACS-2345.) Their literature is a kind of basic, illuminating course about not only colon and rectal cancer but other kinds as well. They also included a booklet from the National Institutes of Health (of which they are an arm) that describes radiation therapy.

Another part of their organization is the Ostomy Rehabilitation Program of the American Cancer Society, also at the same address with the same phone number, in Atlanta.

However, if you call the National Cancer Institute (1-800-4-CANCER), they will give you the latest information on cancer, new techniques, and community services, etc. This is a time-saver because, as they explained to me, calling the National Institutes of Health (their parent) in Maryland will result in pushing a lot of those telephone buttons we all hate. And the National Institutes really prefer that you call 1-800-4-CANCER. It's quicker and simpler.

The National Cancer Institute also has a publications ordering service, which will send information on almost anything you request. Their address is P.O. Box 24128, Baltimore, Maryland 21227.

The United Ostomy Association, Inc. [36 Executive Park, Suite 120, Irvine, California 92614-6744. Phone: 1-800-826-0826, Fax: (714) 660-9262], is a great source for help. One of their booklets, for instance, is *Sex, Pregnancy and the Female Ostomate*. They will give you the names and locations of chapters in your area. What do these chapters do? They will, in addition to providing information, inform you of meetings, events, lectures, and conventions that will introduce you to other people who have had the same procedure as you are going to have. At gatherings you will be shown the latest in medical supplies, and you will be able to talk with experts in the field. The Ostomy Association has volunteers who will come and share their own experiences, particularly when you are just beginning to recover and need all the advice and support you can get. They also publish *Ostomy Quarterly*, for a separate fee, which is bright, upbeat, and informative.

I have to admit, however, they are very hard to get on the phone. Be persistent, keep calling, and leave your message on their voice mails. Once you receive their application for membership and mail it back, they will bill you later. Dues are based on your local chapter.

The WCET—World Council of Enterostomal Therapists [P.O. Box 48099, 60 Dundas Street East, Mississauga, Ontario, L5A 468, Canada. Phone: (905) 848-9400]—is another group to contact. Although I have never spoken to them, they are on Terry Haus's recommended list of places to call. They are able to give you the name of E.T. nurses all over the world. For instance, if you are about to travel, it would be a good idea to call them for their list. Then, if you experience an emergency in any country, you would have the name of a professional to contact.

The WOCN—Wound Ostomy Conference Nurses, Association of Enterostomal Therapy Nurses [1550 S. Coast Highway, Suite 201, Laguna Beach, California 92651. Phone: (888) 224-WOCN]—can help you contact, even in small or rural areas, nurses who can give you preop counseling and instruction. With advance notice, the doctor can arrange for an E.T. nurse to meet you in his office before the surgery. Later, when your doctor has necessarily gone on to the next case, it is a particular comfort to have access to a nurse who might visit your house and lead you through the difficult steps of healing, care, and irrigation.

In England there is the International Ostomy Association—IOA (15 Station Road, Reading, Berkshire RG1 1LG, England. Phone: 44-1-734-391537, Fax: 734-569-095). Howard Jones is in charge here, so ask for him. The IOA will put you in touch with lay persons, support groups, and referrals for almost every area in Europe. They may give you the name and number of the local support group leader. If you need help, they will,

Sources

for example, put you in touch with an ostomate who could help you find whatever you need in whatever city or country you happen to be.

Terry Haus tells me that if you experience difficulty in any foreign country and you have no phone numbers, go directly to a teaching hospital. "It might not be the fanciest hospital," she said, "but they may know, more than any other place, what to do, and they may even have the supplies you need, although that is not always the case."

I was very lucky to have Terry Haus come into my life. It was her kind of dedication and knowledge that really made me able to bear the struggle it took to get well. (One of her male, Hasidic patients, who ordinarily cannot be touched by a woman not in his family, calls her "an angel.") She informs me that many hospitals are doing away with their ostomy specialists for budgetary reasons. This is a terrible tragedy because their compassion and know-how are life-saving. If your hospital does not have an ostomy specialist, please urge them—*beg* them—to hire one. And do contact the above sources as well.

Index

Index

Index

Index

technique of, 216–18, 220–25
traveling and, 225

Jackson, Dr., 189–91

Kahn, Dr., 61
Keith, Larry, 193–201, 209
Kelly, Dr. John, 59–73, 82, 95–99,
    103–5, 107, 110, 118–19,
    165–67, 187–88
  herniated colostomy repair by,
    173–81, 184–85
  removal of Barbara's stitches by,
    138–41
Kennedy, Jacqueline, 125
Kimberg-Kern, Allison, 229
Klugman, Jack, 218
Kramer, Dr. Jeffrey, 85–87, 148, 196,
    198–99, 237–39
Kucynski, Charlotte, 55–56, 58,
    218–19

Ladies Home Journal, 100, 226
Lamb, Wendy, 19
Landis, Scott, 19–20, 168–69
Lang, Fritz, 32
Lapine, Caroline, 137
Leigh, Bobbie, 103–4, 157
Leigh, John, 103–4
Lesane, Katherine, 186–88
Levy, Dr. Joseph, 17
Life Force, The (Shaw), 122
Living Wills, 124
London, 22–28
  rehearsals for *Scarlett* in,
    24–28
Lopez, Rosa, 210–11
lymph nodes, 97, 101, 105

Ma, Yo-Yo, 158
McCarthy, Charlie, 67
McClanahan, Rue, 192–201, 228
MacMillan, Dr., 179–80
Maggie (nurse), 119–22
  and murder of son, 120–22
Mairs, Nancy, 239
Manhattan Theatre Club, 168, 172,
    200, 214
Masur, Kurt, 74
Meara, Anne, 168, 192–201, 228
Mears, Dr. J. Gregory, 106–7, 139,
    152, 161, 185–88, 213, 231–32,
    233–36

bedside manner of, 107, 145
  career of, 235–36
Meisenheimer, Edwin, 51
Merwin, W. S., 22, 242
Metropolitan Museum of Art, 16–18,
    229
Midsummer Night's Dream, A (Shake-
    speare), 39
Moreau, Jeanne, 27
M.O.S. ("mid-out sound"), 32
Mozart, Wolfgang Amadeus, 167,
    243
Museum of Modern Art, 16
My Breast (television movie), 96

National Cancer Institute,
    248–50
National Institutes of Health, 245
New York, 63
New York, N.Y., west side of, 18–19,
    74–75
New York Philharmonic, 74
New York University Medical Cen-
    ter, 49–52, 191, 202–6
  Barbara's second colostomy at,
    215–19
Nichols, Mike, 196–97
No Exit (Sartre), 100
nurses:
  chemotherapy, 229–30
  ostomy, 217–18
  see also Doris; Haus, Terry;
    Maggie

O'Connell, Tim, 13
Oliver, Rochelle, 192–201, 207
oncologists, 97
  see also Anderson, Dr.; Mears, Dr.
    J. Gregory
One Potato, Two Potato (film), 110
ostomates, ostomy, 88, 112–17
  see also Haus, Terry; nurses,
    ostomy
Ostomy Society, 250
ostomy support groups, 136–37

Papp, Joseph, 117
patients, proactive vs. passive,
    234–35
Patrimony (Roth), 213
Perlberger, Carol, 53–54
Peterson, Oscar, 240
Pogrebin, Bert, 103

Index